MIDWIFERY

Medical Conditions

For Elsevier

Content Strategist: Alison Taylor
Content Development Specialist: Veronika Watkins
Project Manager: Julie Taylor
Designer: Paula Catalano
Illustration Manager: Paula Catalano

VOLUME **8**

MIDWIFERY ESSENTIALS

Medical Conditions

Helen Baston, BA(Hons), MMedSci, PhD, PGDipEd, ADM, RN, RM
Consultant Midwife Public Health; Sheffield Teaching Hospitals NHS
Foundation Trust, UK; Honorary Researcher/Lecturer, University of
Sheffield; Honorary Lecturer Sheffield Hallam University, UK

Jenny Hall, EdD, MSc, RN, RM, ADM, PGDip(HE) SFHEA, FRCM
Independent Midwifery Educator and Researcher, Bristol, UK

Jayne Samples, DM, MSc, BSc(Hons), RM, RGN, FHEA
Senior Lecturer in Midwifery, Lead Midwife for Education,
Department of Nursing and Midwifery,
University of Huddersfield, UK

ELSEVIER

Edinburgh London New York Oxford Philadelphia St Louis Sydney Toronto 2019

Notices

Practitioners and researchers must always rely on their own experience and knowledge in evaluating and using any information, methods, compounds or experiments described herein. Because of rapid advances in the medical sciences, in particular, independent verification of diagnoses and drug dosages should be made. To the fullest extent of the law, no responsibility is assumed by Elsevier, authors, editors or contributors for any injury and/or damage to persons or property as a matter of products liability, negligence or otherwise, or from any use or operation of any methods, products, instructions, or ideas contained in the material herein.

ISBN 978-0-7020-7104-1
e_ISBN 978-0-7020-7160-7

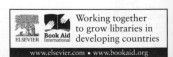

Printed in China

Contents

Preface

To contribute to the provision of sensitive, safe and effective maternity care for women and their families is a privilege. Childbirth is a life-changing event for women. Those around them and those who have an input into any aspect of pregnancy, labour, birth or the postnatal period can positively influence how this event is experienced and perceived. In order to achieve this, maternity carers continually need to reflect on the services they provide and strive to keep up-to-date with developments in clinical practice. They should endeavour to ensure that women are central to the decisions made and that real choices are offered and supported by skilled practitioners.

This book is the eighth volume in a series of texts based on the popular 'Midwifery Basics' series published in *The Practising Midwife* journal. The books have remained true to the original style of the articles and have been updated and expanded to create a user-friendly source of information. They are also intended to stimulate debate and require the reader both to reflect on their current practice, local policies and procedures and to challenge care that is not woman-centred. The use of scenarios enables the practitioner to understand the context of maternity care and explore their role in its safe and effective provision.

There are many dimensions to the provision of woman-centred care that practitioners need to consider and understand. To aid this process, a jigsaw model has been introduced, with the aim of encouraging the reader to explore maternity care from a wide range of perspectives. For example, how does a midwife obtain consent from a woman for a procedure, maintain a safe environment during the delivery of care and make the most of the opportunity to promote health? What are the professional and legal issues in relation to the procedure, and is this practice based on the best available evidence? Which members of the multi-professional team contribute to this aspect of care, and how is it influenced by the way care is organized? Each aspect of the jigsaw should be considered during the assessment, planning, implementation and evaluation of woman-centred maternity care.

Midwifery Essentials: Medical Conditions is about the provision of safe and effective care for women who have or develop illnesses or disabilities whilst pregnant. It reflects the focus of the National Maternity Review publication, *Better Births* (2016), endorsing personalized care and real choice for women. It comprises 10 chapters, each written to stand alone or be read in succession. The introductory chapter sets the scene, exploring the role of the midwife in the context of professional and national guidance. The jigsaw model for midwifery care is introduced and explained, providing a framework to explore each aspect of maternity care, described in subsequent chapters. Chapter 2 explores the principles and practice of caring for women who have cancer and the impact of this on their emotional and social wellbeing. Chapter 3 focuses on the care of women who have a hypertensive disorder, and Chapter 4 considers how respiratory illnesses create challenges for the mother-to-be. Chapter 5 focuses on blood disorders, and Chapter 6 describes digestive illnesses and how they can be managed throughout pregnancy. In Chapter 7 a range of cardiac conditions are explored to provide insight into why this is now the leading cause of indirect maternal death in the UK. Chapter 8 focuses on the significance of chronic infections, such as hepatitis and HIV, and Chapter 9 looks at how neurological conditions can be safely managed. The book concludes with Chapter 10, which describes the impact of endocrine conditions on women during pregnancy and childbirth. This book thoroughly prepares the reader to provide safe, evidence-based, woman-centred care for mothers whose pregnancies are shaped by a medical condition or chronic disability.

National Maternity Review (2016) Better Births. Improving outcomes of maternity services in England. Available at: https://www.england.nhs.uk/wp-content/uploads/2016/02/national-maternity-review-report.pdf

Sheffield, Bristol and Huddersfield 2019

Helen Baston
Jennifer Hall
Jayne Samples

Acknowledgements

In the process of writing, there are always people behind the scenes who support or add to the development of the book. We would specifically like to thank Mary Seager, formerly Senior Commissioning Editor at Elsevier, for her initial vision, support and prompting to turn the journal articles from *The Practising Midwife* into a readable volume. This project has now further developed with the insight and patience of Veronika Watkins and Alison Taylor. In addition, neither of us could have completed this edition without the love, support and endless patience of our amazing families. To you we owe our greatest gratitude.

Contributors

Rachel Jokhi, MEd, FHEA, PGDip, BA(Hons), RM
Midwifery Teacher, Lead Midwife for Education, Deputy Director of
 Learning and Teaching, University of Sheffield, Sheffield, UK

Roobin Jokhi, BMedSci(Hons), MBChB, MRCOG, MD
Consultant Obstetrician, Maternal and Fetal Medicine Specialist,
 Sheffield Teaching Hospitals NHSFT, Honorary Lecturer,
 University of Sheffield, Sheffield, UK

CHAPTER 1

Introduction

This book is the eighth in the *Midwifery Essentials* series aimed at student midwives and those who support them in clinical practice. It focuses on medical conditions and how they might impact on the woman's experience of pregnancy. Scenarios are used throughout the book to facilitate learning and assist the reader to apply this knowledge to their own practice areas. The focus for contemporary maternity care is choice and continuity of care within a safe and personalized service (National Maternity Review 2016). The aim of this book is to explore ways in which this aspiration can become a reality for women and their families, despite the complexities of their condition.

Social and psychological impact of medical conditions

The changing demographics of women embarking on pregnancy is having an impact on the number who have a known medical condition. Between 2001 and 2017 the number of women having a baby in their forties has risen 80% (Royal College of Midwives (RCM) 2018) with the increased likelihood of these women requiring support for potential medical conditions. In addition, in the population globally, fewer women have a healthy weight, with over a third being overweight or clinically obese (World Health Organization 2016). This situation has led to rising rates of conditions such as diabetes and heart disease and effects on other parts of the body.

The increasing rates of medical conditions lead to greater need within the maternity services for specialist care. Though midwives may remain as the lead carer, the majority of women will also require support and assessment from a variety of members of the multi-disciplinary team. For women, this will incur a cost of stress and anxiety related to additional clinic appointments and tests.

For many women this pregnancy will also be an investment emotionally. Whilst for some, pregnancy will be welcome, as they have waited for and been through tests and processes to become pregnant, there may also be anxiety related to fears of losing the baby or around the impact on their health condition. There is a known connection between long-term medical conditions and mental wellbeing (RCPSych n.d.). It is suggested that previous medical conditions in pregnancy contribute to higher levels of psychosocial stress in pregnancy (Melville et al 2010). However, it will also be the case that psychosocial stress will be increased when a condition is diagnosed or becomes worse during pregnancy.

The midwife's role in all these circumstances should be recognizing a woman's and her family's needs holistically. Midwives and other carers in pregnancy need to be aware of the mental health needs of all women, particularly those coping with ongoing or new health conditions. When reading the following chapters of the book consider how a woman may be feeling while going through the tests, investigations and appointments associated with her conditions and how any additional stress may be alleviated.

The aim of this introductory chapter is to introduce the 'jigsaw model' for exploring effective midwifery practice.

The jigsaw model (Fig. 1.1) is used throughout the book, with a view to helping midwives apply their knowledge to the provision of woman-centred maternity care.

Midwifery care model

One of the purposes of this series is to consider the care of women and their babies from a holistic viewpoint. This means considering the care from a physical, emotional, psychological, spiritual, social and cultural context. To do this we have devised a jigsaw model of care that will encourage the reader to consider individual aspects of care, while

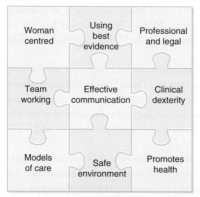

Fig. 1.1 Jigsaw model: dimensions of effective midwifery care.

recognizing that these aspects go to make up part of the whole person being cared for.

This model will be used to reflect on the clinical scenarios described in the chapters. It shows the dimensions for effective maternity care, and each should be considered during the assessment, planning, implementation and evaluation of an aspect of care.

The pieces of the jigsaw (see Fig. 1.1) clearly interlink with each other, and each is needed for the provision of safe, holistic care. When one is missing, the picture will be incomplete and care will not reach its potential. Each aspect of the model is described next in more detail. It is recommended that when an aspect of midwifery care is being evaluated, each piece of the jigsaw is addressed. Consider the questions pertaining to each piece of the jigsaw, and work through those that are relevant to the clinical situation you face.

Woman-centred care

The provision of woman-centred care was one of the central messages of the policy document *Changing Childbirth* (Department of Health 1993), which turned the focus of maternity care from meeting the needs of professionals to listening and responding to the aspirations of women. This was further enforced in the *National Service Framework* (Department of Health 2004) and *Maternity Matters* (Department of Health 2007) and reflected in *Better Births* (National Maternity Review 2016). The provision of woman-centred care is also reflected in an expectation of the National Institute for Health and Care Excellence ((NICE) 2008, 2017) and is an expectation of midwifery practice highlighted in pre-registration education (Nursing and Midwifery Council (NMC) 2009). When considering particular aspects of care, the questions that need to be addressed to ensure that the woman's care is woman-centred include:

- Was the woman involved in the development of her care plan and its subsequent implementation?
- Should her family or carers also be involved?
- How can I ensure that she remains involved in further decisions about her care?
- What are the implications of undertaking or not undertaking this procedure on this particular woman or baby?
- Are there any factors that I need to consider that might influence the results of this procedure for this woman and their impact on her?
- How does this procedure fit in with the woman's hopes, expectations and meanings?
- Is now the most appropriate time to undertake this procedure?

Using best evidence

A growing body of research evidence is available to inform the post-natal care we provide. We have a duty to apply this knowledge, as the NMC Code states: 'always practice in line with the best available evidence' (NMC 2015:7). The use of evidence in practice is complex and multi-faceted, and its application is influenced by many factors, including its authority and consensus amongst colleagues (Kennedy et al 2012).

Questions that need to be addressed when exploring the evidence base of care include:

+ What is already known about this aspect of care?
+ What is the justification for the choices made about care?
+ What research evidence is available on this procedure/test?
+ Do local guidelines reflect best evidence?
+ Was a midwife involved in the development of local/national guidelines?
+ Who represents users of maternity services on groups where guidelines are developed?
+ What midwifery research project has your trust been involved in?
+ Where do you go first in order to identify sources of best evidence?

Professional and legal

Women need to feel confident that the midwives who care for them are working within a framework that supports safe practice. Midwives who practise in the United Kingdom must adhere to the guidance of the NMC. The Code (NMC 2015:02) states:

> UK nurses and midwives must act in line with the Code, whether they are providing direct care to individuals, groups or communities or bringing their professional knowledge to bear on nursing and midwifery practice in other roles, such as leadership, education or research. This commitment to professional standards is fundamental to being part of a profession.

Midwives are therefore required to comply with English law and the rules and regulations of their employers.

Questions that need to be addressed to ensure that the woman's care fulfils statutory obligations include:

+ Is this procedure expected to be an integral part of education before qualification?
+ Which NMC proficiencies relate to this care/test?
+ How does the NMC Code relate to this care/test?

+ Is any other NMC guidance applicable to this care/test?
+ Are there any national or international guidelines for this care/test?
+ Are there any legal issues underpinning the use of this care/test?

Team working

Whilst midwives are the experts in low-risk antenatal care, they remain reliant on a number of other workers to provide a comprehensive, safe service. Midwives work as part of a team of professionals who each bring particular skills and perspectives to the care of women and their families. The NMC Code requires registrants to 'support students' and colleagues' learning to help them develop their professional competence and confidence' (2015:9). It also states:

+ Respect the skills, expertise and contributions of your colleagues, referring matters to them when appropriate
+ Maintain effective communication with colleagues
+ Keep colleagues informed when you are sharing the care of individuals with other healthcare professionals and staff
+ Work with colleagues to evaluate the quality of your work and that of the team
+ Work with colleagues to preserve the safety of those receiving care
+ Share information to identify and reduce risk, and
+ Be supportive of colleagues who are encountering health or performance problems. However, this support must never compromise or be at the expense of patient or public safety (NMC 2015:8)

Questions that need to be addressed to ensure that the woman's care makes appropriate use of the multi-professional team include:

+ Does this test fall within my role?
+ Have I acknowledged the limitations of my professional knowledge?
+ Who else will need to be involved to interpret the results?
+ Where should these results be recorded for all to see?
+ Who will I involve if the results are outside normal parameters?
+ How can I facilitate effective team working for this woman?
+ Will another person be required to assist with this care?
+ When will they be available, and how can I access them?

Effective communication

Central to any interaction between a woman and the midwife is effective communication. It is essential that the midwife is aware of the cues she is giving to the woman during the care she provides. Time is often pressured in midwifery, both in the community and hospital setting, but it is important to convey to the woman that she is the focus of your attention. Taking time to explain what you are going to do, and why, is crucial if she is going to trust that you are acting in her best interest. Questions that need to be addressed to ensure that effective communication is achieved before, during and after any aspect of antenatal care include:

+ What information needs to be given in order for the woman to know whether this is the right decision for her?
+ Has she given consent?
+ Is she clear what the care/test entails?
+ In what ways could the information be given?
+ What should be said during the care/test?
+ What should be observed in the woman's behaviour during the care/test?
+ What should be communicated to the woman after the care/test?
+ How and where should recording of the care/test and its results be made?

Clinical dexterity

Midwifery is a profession that requires the practitioner to have a range of knowledge and a repertoire of clinical skills. The midwife continues to learn new skills throughout her working life and is accountable for maintaining and developing her practice as new ways of working are introduced: 'keep your knowledge and skills up to date, taking part in appropriate and regular learning and professional development activities that aim to maintain and develop your competence and improve your performance' (NMC 2015:17).

Questions that need to be addressed to ensure that the woman's care is provided with clinical dexterity include:

+ How has practice changed since I started my education programme/qualified as a midwife?
+ Can I practise this skill in other ways?
+ How has my previous experience influenced how I approach this procedure today?
+ How can I be sure I am carrying this out correctly?
+ Are there opportunities for practising this skill elsewhere?
+ Who can I observe to explore alternative ways of doing this?

Models of care

A midwife works in many settings and in a range of maternity care systems. For example, she may work independently providing holistic client-centred care, or she may work within a large tertiary centre providing care for women with specific health needs. The models of care can be influential in determining the care that a woman may receive, who from and when. Midwives need to consider the most appropriate ways that care can be delivered so that they can influence future development in the best interests of women and their families.

Questions that need to be addressed to ensure that the impact of the way that care is provided is acknowledged include:

+ How long has care been provided in this way?
+ How is the maternity service organized?
+ Which professional groups are involved in the provision of this service?
+ How is this procedure/care influenced by the model of care provided?
+ How does this model of care impact on the carers?
+ How does this model of care impact on the woman and her family?
+ Is this the best way to provide care from a professional point of view?

Safe environment

Midwives providing maternity care need to ensure that the environment in which they work supports safe and effective working practices and protects the woman and her family from harm. The NMC Code states that 'you must maintain the knowledge and skills for safe and effective practice' (NMC 2015:7). The midwife must ensure that the care she gives does not compromise the safety of women and their families. She must therefore create and maintain a safe working environment at all times, whether in a woman's home, a midwifery-led unit or a tertiary maternity service.

Questions that need to be addressed to ensure that the woman's care is provided in a safe environment include:

+ Can the woman be assured that her confidentiality will be maintained?
+ Does the woman understand the implications of giving her consent to this procedure?
+ Are there facilities to ensure that her privacy and dignity are maintained?
+ Is there somewhere to wash hands?
+ Is there an appropriate place to dispose of waste?
+ Is the equipment appropriately maintained and free from contamination?
+ Is the space adequate to allow ease of movement around the woman without invading her personal space?
+ What risks are involved in this procedure/care, and how have they been addressed?
+ Are there any risks to the person undertaking this procedure/care?
+ Is this environment safe for others who might come into the room?

Promotes health

Providing care for women and their families presents a unique opportunity to influence the health and wellbeing of the public. Midwives must capitalize on their contacts with women to help them achieve a healthy pregnancy and birth and promote lifestyle choices that will benefit women, babies and families in the future.

Questions that need to be addressed to ensure that the woman's care promotes health include:

- Is this procedure/care going to help her or harm her or her baby in any way?
- What are the opportunities to use this procedure to educate her/her family on healthy behaviours?
- What resources can women and families access to help them make healthy lifestyle choices?
- Has enough time been allocated to this aspect of care to make the most of the opportunities to promote healthy living?
- Who else should I involve to ensure that the woman and her family get the best possible advice in this situation?

The models of care available and accessed by women can have a significant influence on her experience of pregnancy. The following chapters use the jigsaw model to explore scenarios from practice. Thus the reader is provided with a structure with which to reflect on her care and that of the multi-professional team in which she works. Each chapter includes a range of activities designed to enable the midwife to contextualize the information within her own practice, applying her continually developing knowledge to her own circumstances. The chapters are written so that they can be accessed without having read the previous ones, although we hope you will find the whole book relevant and thought provoking. Enjoy!

References

Department of Health, 1993. Changing Childbirth: Report of the Expert Maternity Group Pt. II; Report of the Expert Maternity Group Pt. 1. Department of Health, London.

Department of Health, 2004. National Service Framework for Children, Young People and Maternity Services. Standard 11. Maternity Services. Department of Health, London.

Department of Health, 2007. Maternity Matters: Choice, Access and Continuity of Care in a Safe Service. Department of Health, London.

Kennedy, H., Doig, E., Hackley, B., et al., 2012. "The midwifery two-step": a study on evidence-based midwifery practice. J. Midwifery Womens Health 57 (5), 454–460.

Melville, J.L., Gavin, A., Guo, Y., et al., 2010. Depressive disorders during pregnancy: prevalence and risk factors in a large urban sample. Obstet. Gynecol. 116 (5), 1064–1070.

National Institute for Health and Care Excellence (NICE 2008, updated 2017) Antenatal care: for uncomplicated pregnancies. CG62. https://www.nice.org.uk/guidance/cg62.

National Maternity Review (2016). Better Births. Improving outcomes of maternity services in England. Available at: https://www.england.nhs.uk/wp-content/uploads/2016/02/national-maternity-review-report.pdf.

Nursing and Midwifery Council (2009). Standards for pre-registration midwifery education. https://www.nmc.org.uk/standards-for-midwives/additional-standards/standards-for-pre-registration-midwifery-education/.

Nursing and Midwifery Council (2015). The code: professional standards of practice and behaviour for nurses and midwives. https://www.nmc.org.uk/globalassets/sitedocuments/nmc-publications/nmc-code.pdf.

RCM 2018 State of Maternity Services report 2018 England https://www.rcm.org.uk/sites/default/files/ENGLAND%20SOMS%202018%20-%20FINAL%20%2803.09.2018%29.pdf.

WHO 2016 Global Health Observatory data 2016 http://www.who.int/gho/ncd/risk_factors/overweight/en/.

CHAPTER 2

Cancer in pregnancy

TRIGGER SCENARIO

Claire came out of the shower with her heart pounding. She quickly dried herself and went and sat on her bed. She gingerly ran her fingers over the spot on her left breast where she thought she had felt a lump. There was no doubt – there it was. She fumbled for her phone and with hands shaking, rang her mum who said, 'Are you sure, love? You know your boobs do change when you are pregnant.'

Introduction

Cancer in pregnancy is rare, although it was the cause of 8% of indirect deaths and 24% of coincidental deaths in women between 6 weeks and 1 year of birth in the UK from 2012–2015 (Knight et al 2017). Increasing maternal age is likely to increase the incidence of cancer diagnosis in childbearing women (Davison et al 2017). There is potential for cancer to develop anywhere in the body. For the purpose of this chapter, the general principles of screening, diagnosis and treatment of cancer will be described, followed by a more detailed exploration of the most common cancers in pregnancy. The importance of multi-professional care and collaboration will be highlighted, as well as the need to involve the woman and her family in the decisions about treatment options throughout her care. Treatment options will be tailored to the individual circumstances of each woman, including the gestation at diagnosis, her aspirations for parenthood and the nature and stage of her cancer.

Preventing cancer

There are many public health campaigns about the benefits of healthy lifestyles, such as stopping smoking (Public Health England (PHE) 2018), for reducing our risk of cancer. Pregnancy provides another opportunity for health professionals to discuss the importance of these messages not only for helping grow a healthy baby but also for keeping the family in optimum health in years to come. It is also important to convey the value of childbearing-related practices that can also help reduce the risk of cancers in women.

For example, continuous breastfeeding prevents ovulation, which in turn reduces a woman's exposure to oestrogens, which are linked to development of breast and ovarian cancer. A study exploring the economic benefits of breastfeeding demonstrated that if women who choose to breastfeed do so for longer, the health benefits this could bring would reap savings of millions of pounds, as well as impact on quality of life (Pokhrel et al 2015).

Activity

Read the paper 'Preventing Disease and Saving Resources' (Renfrew et al 2012). Consider the impact of breastfeeding on the health of the baby, neonate, child and adult. How might you convey these messages to women in your care?

Activity

Are boys offered human papilloma virus (HPV) vaccination? What cancers is HPV linked to? Can adults receive the HPV vaccination?

Screening for cancer

Currently three cancer screening programmes are available to women in the UK (Table 2.1). Screening involves testing apparently healthy people for signs of a disease (Cancer Research UK 2018), but it will not identify all cancers. However, screening is not without its risks; for example, it is known that some cancers identified through mammography will be treated that might not have ever caused symptoms. But it will identify some cancers that would not have been detected through self-examination and therefore, on balance, is routinely offered to women who are most at risk from 50 years of age. Cervical screening can identify cells that might suggest a cervical abnormality. Not all require treatment, and even if treatment is required, most do not develop into cancer (TOMBOLA Group 2009).

Diagnosing cancer

Building up a picture from a range of sources is how a cancer diagnosis is often made. Symptoms may have been vague and quite general in the

Table 2.1: **Cancer screening programmes UK**

Cancer	Screening method
Breast	Self-examination Mammography routinely offered between ages 50 and 70 years every 3 years
Cervical	Smear routinely offered between ages 25 and 64 years every 3 years
Bowel	Age 55 years: bowel scope screening Age 60–74: home testing for blood in faeces every 2 years

Table 2.2: **Signs and symptoms of some common cancers**

Type of cancer	Signs/symptoms	Additional information
Breast	Lump or thickening Puckering of the skin Discharge from the nipple	Family history Previous lumpectomy Obesity Oral contraceptives Alcohol
Cervical	Abnormal vaginal bleeding Vaginal discharge Pain during sex Back or pelvic pain	Family history Previous abnormal smear History of HPV infection Smoking
Lung	Persistent cough Breathlessness Haemoptysis	Smoker/ex-smoker Exposure to pollutants Family history
Colon	Blood in stools Change in bowel motions	Previous history of polyps History of Crohn's disease Family history
Blood	Fatigue Breathlessness Bruising	Exposure to radiation, benzene Chemotherapy Smoking Family history

first instance but become more specific and persistent with time. Many people have a 'wait and see' approach to any out-of-the-ordinary changes to their health, but as methods of cancer diagnosis become more sophisticated and early treatment outcomes become more effective, many public health campaigns encourage us to seek advice sooner rather than later.

In the UK, the first medical point of contact will be the individual's general practitioner (GP). The GP is well placed to put any new symptoms into the context of the person's previous medical, family and current health history. See Table 2.2 for a summary of some signs and symptoms of common cancers.

Access the National Institute for Health and Care Excellence (NICE) Guideline NG12 – Suspected cancer: recognition and referral (*https:// www.nice.org.uk/guidance/ng12*).

Look at the recommendations for referral when breast, ovarian or skin cancer is suspected.

Current health history

Many people in the early stages of cancer will feel quite well and not experience any changes in their general wellbeing. However, for some, it may be that their energy levels are reduced or they experience some weight loss, breathlessness or pain which prompts them to seek advice. It may be a combination of factors that alerts the GP to think 'could this be cancer', especially when there are red flag signs as well as general symptoms of malaise, such as intermenstrual bleeding, detection of a lump or abnormal appearance of skin lesions.

Physical examination

Depending on the symptoms reported, a general or more specific physical examination will be conducted by the GP. This will include baseline observations such as temperature, heart rate and blood pressure, followed by auscultating chest and heart sounds. Examination of axilla and neck lymph nodes will also be undertaken, especially when a history of fatigue is given.

If a gynaecological cancer is suspected following a relevant health history, a pelvic examination may be undertaken by the doctor, who will also palpate lymph nodes for enlargement. An abdominal examination for palpable masses or organ enlargement will be performed where symptoms of abdominal pain, bloating and dyspepsia are reported. A digital rectal examination (DRE) might be indicated if rectal bleeding is reported. A neurological examination (see Chapter 9) will be undertaken where there is a history of headaches, dizziness or visual disturbance.

Symptoms in pregnancy

As can be seen in Table 2.2, a number of potential cancer signs and symptoms might be present that are actually common in pregnancy – see Table 2.3 for some examples. It is therefore paramount that even seemingly small signs and symptoms disclosed during pregnancy are clearly documented and followed up and referral sought where persistent.

Table 2.3: **Pregnancy explanations for common cancer symptoms**

Cancer symptoms	Pregnancy explanation
Breast changes, discomfort, discharging nipple	Breast enlargement, pigmentation, stretch marks, colostrum production
Fatigue	Anaemia, haemodilution
Breathlessness	Anaemia, growing uterus
Abdominal pain	Stretching ligaments, Braxton-Hicks
Backache	Lax ligaments, postural
Headache	Tension, stress, pre-eclampsia
Nausea and vomiting	'Morning' sickness, hyperemesis gravidarum
Constipation	Impact of progesterone
Vaginal bleeding (pv)	Threatened miscarriage, possible antepartum haemorrhage
Rectal bleeding (pr)	haemorrhoids

Table 2.4: **Common diagnostic tests for cancer**

Location	Diagnosis
Breast	MRI, ultrasound, biopsy
Cervical	Colposcopy and biopsy, computed tomography (CT) scan, MRI, positron emission tomography (PET), ultrasound
Colon	Colonoscopy and biopsy, blood tests, CT scan, ultrasound
Melanoma	Dermoscopy; punch, scrape or excision biopsy
Leukaemia	Blood tests, bone marrow biopsy, lumbar puncture

Diagnostic tests

Many tests are used for diagnosing cancer, its type and its spread. One test may lead to another, so the first few days and weeks can be a roller coaster of 'appointment–test–result–appointment–test–result' until a clear picture is developed of the nature of the cancer and the most appropriate programme of treatment. See Table 2.4 for a summary of some of the most common tests.

Activity

Access *https://www.cancerresearchuk.org/about-cancer/cancer-in-general/tests*.

Look up some of the tests that you are not familiar with. Read about what the test will involve for the patient so that you have an understanding of what they might be going through.

Treating cancer in pregnancy

From a medical point of view, the woman's life and saving or prolonging it is paramount. However, many women with a cancer diagnosis in pregnancy elect to continue with the pregnancy and sometimes delay treatment. These decisions can be heart-breaking for families, with partners, parents and friends all having a view of the best route to take. Generally speaking, with an aggressive cancer diagnosed in the first trimester, a woman may be offered a medical termination of the pregnancy to enable treatment to begin without delay. She may decide to continue with the pregnancy and start treatment, continue with the pregnancy and wait until the second trimester to start treatment or elect not to have any treatment until after the birth. However, the final choice is hers to make, and both she and her family will need sensitive, empathic care both during the decision-making process and subsequently.

Preserving fertility

Women who are diagnosed with cancer during pregnancy and who want more children in the future may wish to consider the options in relation to fertility preservation. As with all fertility treatments, there is no guarantee that such procedures will lead to a future pregnancy, and options vary depending on what services are locally available.

The options are not without risks themselves and include:

+ Freezing ovarian tissue
* Freezing eggs
+ Freezing embryos
+ Ovarian suppression
* Wait and see

Activity

Find out what fertility treatments are available in your locality. What are the pregnancy success rates following implantation of frozen embryos? What are the risks associated with fertility treatment?

Surgery

Surgery is often the first line of treatment for cancer or is secondary to treatment to reduce a tumour. There are many cases of successful surgical procedures undertaken in pregnancy, and this will depend on the location, gestation, spread and general health of the mother (see Table 2.5 for common medical terminology associated with cancer diagnosis and treatment). The Confidential Enquiry into Maternal Deaths (Knight

Table 2.5: **Common medical terminology**

Term	Meaning
Hysterectomy	Removal of the uterus
Salpingectomy	Removal of a fallopian tube
Oophorectomy	Removal of an ovary
Cystoscopy	Camera inserted into the bladder
Colonoscopy	Camera inserted into the whole colon
Proctoscopy	Camera inserted into the rectum
Sigmoidoscopy	Camera inserted into the lower colon
Haematemesis	Vomiting blood
Haemoptysis	Coughing up blood
Haematuria	Blood in urine
Haematochezia	Blood in stool

et al 2017:v) asserts, 'Pregnancy should not be viewed as a contraindication to surgery in the presence of malignancy'.

Chemotherapy

The cytotoxic agents used during the treatment of cancer pass through the placenta and have the potential to be teratogenic (cause malformations in the embryo or fetus), especially when the organs are being formed between 2 and 8 weeks' gestation (Davison et al 2017). There is no evidence of major malformations in babies of mothers receiving chemotherapy after the first trimester or of childhood impairment in children exposed to cancer and/or chemotherapy (Amant et al 2015). The usual chemotherapy treatment plans (as for non-pregnancy women) should be offered after 14 weeks of pregnancy (Amant et al 2012).

When women are being treated for cancer, there is an increased risk of premature birth, growth restriction and stillbirth. If delayed growth or fetal compromise is detected, then birth is likely to be expedited, following steroid administration to facilitate lung maturity. In the absence of fetal concern, however, iatrogenic preterm birth should be avoided where possible, as it is associated with long-term sequelae for the child, including cognitive impairment (Knight et al 2015).

The woman must be involved in decisions about her care package throughout. The usual treatment plan may be adapted following careful counselling of the apparent risks for each option available and according to her wishes. For example, she may decide to receive single-drug treatment in the first trimester, waiting until the second trimester for the usual multi-drug approach.

Radiation

Based on evidence from studies of cases following exposure to nuclear explosions and X-ray in pregnancy (International Commission on Radiological Protection 2003), it has long been practised that radiation therapy, if indicated during an ongoing pregnancy, should be deferred until after the birth because of the potential impact on the fetus. When exposed in the first trimester, the effects can be childhood cancer development and mental retardation. There is, however, case study evidence (Kal & Struikmans 2005) that when the cancer is remote from the pelvis or where the dose is low and the fetus shielded no ill effects are experienced. There is also some case study evidence of effective treatment for cancer using the alternative carbon-ion therapy during pregnancy that did not result in harm to the fetus (Munter et al 2010).

Thromboprophylaxis

A cancer diagnosis is an independent risk factor for venous thromboembolism (VTE), which continues to the most significant cause of direct maternal death (Knight et al 2017). Hence all women should be assessed for their VTE risk and treated according to the most recent Royal College of Obstetricians and Gynaecologists (RCOG) guideline (RCOG 2015). Care should continue to be coordinated postnatally to ensure there are no contraindications (Knight et al 2015).

Support during treatment

Having treatment for cancer is an emotional journey for any woman, but during pregnancy some of the side effects can be particularly challenging. Fatigue is common in early pregnancy, but exacerbated by a cancer diagnosis, it can be overwhelming. It is made worse by the emotional trauma, frequent attendance for appointments and anticipation of results, as well as the physical side effects of treatment such as nausea and vomiting.

Women should be encouraged to accept all offers of help to enable her to focus on her developing baby or other children. Help with shopping, cooking, cleaning and traveling to appointments are all practical ways that people can contribute. However, it is also vital that women have someone they can confide in regarding their hopes and fears; this may be through the local cancer service, peer support opportunities and the continuity of care given by a named midwife.

Some women may be concerned about becoming too attached to their baby, worrying that the baby might be harmed by any treatment or that they might not be around to see their baby grow up. Encouraging women to talk to their developing baby, keeping a journal about their journey together and expressing any anxieties before they become huge problems can be useful strategies to help her develop a meaningful relationship that will be important to them both, whatever the long-term outcome.

Breast cancer

The incidence of breast cancer in the UK is one in eight women, and it increases with age, with eight out of ten women who develop breast cancer being postmenopausal (Cancer Research UK 2018). Anyone with a diagnosis of breast cancer should receive specialist psychological support and through the support of a named clinical nurse specialist have the opportunity to take part in research (NICE 2009, 2018). Survival rates are good, with 78% of women surviving 10 years or more (Cancer Research UK 2018).

Diagnosis

Magnetic resonance imaging (MRI) uses radio waves and magnetism to create a picture of the body in cross-sectional pictures. Although it is thought to be safe in pregnancy, it is not usually undertaken in the first trimester as a precaution (Cancer Research UK 2017). Fine needle aspiration is not recommended during pregnancy because of the potential for false-positive or false-negative results (Amant et al 2010). A range of treatment options are available depending on the nature and stage of the cancer.

Treatment

Surgery is generally the first line of treatment for breast cancer, and this can take the form of simple lumpectomy or radical mastectomy, where lymph tissue is also taken for histological examination.

> #### Activity
>
> What is tamoxifen? In which types of cancer treatment is it recommended? What are its side effects? What are the recommendations regarding pregnancy and this drug?

Breast cancer in pregnancy

The definition of breast cancer associated with pregnancy is when it is 'diagnosed in pregnancy, breastfeeding or the first year after birth' (Monteiro et al 2013:174). As the incidence of cancer increases with age and the age of childbearing increases, it is likely that an increase in the number of cancers diagnosed in pregnancy will also be seen. There is, however, an increase in the rates of breast cancer in younger women

(Ksheerasagar et al 2017), so although rare in pregnancy, maternity staff should not dismiss the possibility if a woman presents with symptoms.

The incidence of pregnancy-associated breast cancer (PABC) is approximately 1 in 3000 (Navrozoglou et al 2008). The main aim when treating breast cancer is to halt the spread of the disease and to prevent the development of metastatic spread; this should be equally applied during pregnancy as outside of pregnancy.

Surgery can take place at any gestation and should be accompanied by thromboprophylaxis because of the combined risk of pregnancy, surgery and malignancy (Anant et al 2012).

Chemotherapy is generally considered safe during pregnancy, especially if started after the first trimester. It should be avoided, however, in the 3 weeks preceding the birth, where possible, to avoid the added risks of bleeding, infection and anaemia (Anant et al 2012).

It is general practice that radiotherapy be postponed until after the birth, if deemed an appropriate treatment option (Monteiro et al 2013). There is an online tool, 'Predict', (Candido et al 2017) for professionals and patients to use to consider the most appropriate treatment options after surgery, depending on the type of cancer.

Diagnosis of cancer during pregnancy is associated with an increased caesarean section rate and induction of labour (Kent et al 2015). Babies born to mothers with breast cancer are more likely to be born prematurely with all the associated ramifications of low birth weight, respiratory distress syndrome (RDS), jaundice and hypoglycaemia (Kent et al 2015).

The placenta should be sent for histology to look for metastatic changes, and breastfeeding is not recommended following recent chemotherapy (Amant et al 2012).

Cervical cancer

This is the most common cancer in women under 35 years of age with over 3000 women being diagnosed in the UK each year (NHS England 2017). Survival rates are high, with 63% of women diagnosed with cervical cancer surviving for 10 years or more (Cancer Research UK 2018).

Diagnosis

Colposcopy is offered if abnormal cells are identified following a smear or there is a significant history of intermenstrual or postmenopausal bleeding. During this procedure a speculum is inserted into the vagina to enable the doctor to see the cervix and a colposcope used to look for abnormal tissue. This is not usually painful and can be carried out in pregnancy or between periods if not. If such an area is identified, a biopsy will be taken and the sample of tissue sent to the laboratory for histological examination. This aspect can be uncomfortable and cause spotting and cramping.

Treatment

There are a range of options depending on the type of cancer and its spread. These include:

+ Large loop excision of the transformation zone (LLETZ): This uses a loop of wire with an electrical current to remove the tissue in the affected area.
+ Cone biopsy.
+ Surgery: Usually a hysterectomy is performed, although for women who wish to have a baby and the cancer is in its early stages, it may be possible to perform a radical trachelectomy, which preserves enough of the cervix for fertility to be maintained. Lymph nodes may also be removed to test for further spread.
+ Chemotherapy and/or radiotherapy: A combination of drug treatment and radiation is used to shrink the tumour. This can also be used for palliative control of symptoms where the cancer has already spread and cannot be cured.

Cervical cancer and pregnancy

The results of a Cochrane systematic review found that women who have had local treatment for cancer do not have reduced fertility rates compared with untreated women (Kyrgiou et al 2015). However, rates of second-trimester miscarriage and ectopic pregnancies were higher in treated women. There is evidence that the rates of preterm birth are related to the amount of tissue removed (Castanon et al 2014), so there is need for a careful balance between preserving fertility and effective treatment of the cancer.

If a woman is pregnant when cervical cancer is diagnosed and chooses to continue with her pregnancy, multi-disciplinary care should be instigated, with birth after 35 weeks' gestation aimed for if possible (NICE 2017). Caesarean birth is the preferred mode of birth (Zhang et al 2015). Whilst vaginal birth may be achievable, there is the potential added risk of haemorrhage and embolization of the tumour (Samarasinghe & Shafi 2014).

Activity

Access the NICE Clinical Knowledge Summaries for cervical cancer (*https://cks.nice.org.uk/cervical-cancer-and-hpv#!scenario:1*).

Consider the different classifications of cervical cancer and the first-line treatment options.

Lymphoma

This cancer is divided into two groups: Hodgkin's lymphoma (HL) and non-Hodgkin's lymphoma (NHL) (Karen et al 2010). It originates in the lymph glands or other organs of the lymphatic system such as the spleen and bone marrow. Symptoms include:

+ Fever
+ Night sweats
+ Swollen lymph glands
+ Fatigue
+ Weight loss
+ Cough
+ Abdominal distension or pain (Cancer Centre 2018)

Whilst staging of the disease is an important aspect of developing an appropriate treatment plan, the use of invasive procedures and radiation imaging should be used with caution where other methods such as clinical and haematological examination and ultrasound can be employed (Bachanova & Connors 2013). HL is rarely diagnosed in pregnancy (1:6000 births), but because treatments are effective and less toxic, more women are surviving HL and becoming pregnant where the condition may relapse (George-Carey et al 2017). Multi-professional team care is paramount to ensure the most effective care and management of the condition.

> ### Activity
>
> What is meant by 'B symptoms'? What is meant by the terms *anaemia*, *leucopoenia* and *thrombocytopaenia*? What blood tests are recommended when lymphoma is suspected?

Leukaemia

This is a cancer in which there is an over-production of immature white blood cells (blasts) leading to a decrease in the number of red blood cells and platelets. Thus the ability to fight infection is reduced coupled with anaemia and risk of bleeding.

Diagnosis of leukaemia in pregnancy is rare, at approximately 1 in 75,000 pregnancies, and most of these are the acute form (Ali et al 2015). The impact of the disease on the outcome of pregnancy is significant, including miscarriage and fetal growth restriction (Chelghoum et al 2005). The risk of maternal death from the disease is such that treatment should not be delayed, and this has implications for continuation of the pregnancy. It is thought that if diagnosed in the first trimester, elective termination of pregnancy is safer for the mother than the risk to her of spontaneous miscarriage and subsequent bleeding, as haemostasis could be controlled more effectively in the former situation (Ali et al 2015). The impact of chemotherapy treatment on the fetus in the second and third trimesters is an increased risk of prematurity, sepsis and growth restriction, yet there is the need to start treatment as soon as possible for the best maternal outcomes. Hence, all decisions and options should be carefully considered in discussion with the woman and the obstetric and medical teams.

Women who have leukaemia are at increased risk of sepsis, and her care team should be alert to the signs of infection and situations that might increase her exposure to infection, such as ruptured membranes and induction of labour. Antibiotics and anti-fungal agents may be used prophylactically as well as therapeutically (Ali et al 2015).

Activity

What is myeloma? Find out what is known about the prognosis for acute myeloblastic leukaemia and acute lymphoblastic leukaemia.

Melanoma

Malignant melanoma (MM) is one of the most common cancers affecting young women, and about one-third of all MM diagnoses are in women of childbearing age (Bradford et al 2010). Following a review of the limited available evidence to date, there is currently no indication for delaying or ending pregnancies in women with early-stage disease, and there is no evidence that pregnancy impacts on its prognosis (Todd & Driscoll 2017). MRI scan may be used for staging the disease in the second and third trimesters (Patenaude et al 2014), and surgical excision should not be postponed (Walker et al 2016).

Examination of the placenta should be part of the pathway of care for women with this disease. In a review of the studies exploring fetal metastasis or placental involvement (Alexander et al 2003) MM was the most prevalent cancer leading to such spread (40% involved the fetus and 31% the placenta).

Gestational trophoblastic disease

This disease group is made up of benign and invasive moles, choriocarcinoma and trophoblastic tumours (Table 2.6).

Table 2.6: **Gestational trophoblastic diseases**

Group	Type	Incidence
Premalignant	Partial hydatidiform mole	1 per 100 pregnancies
	Complete hydatidiform mole	1–2 per 1000 pregnancies
Malignant gestational trophoblastic neoplasia (GTN)	Invasive mole	2% of pregnancies with partial hydatidiform mole
	Gestational choriocarcinoma	15%–20% of pregnancies with complete hydatidiform mole (Hermandez 2018)
	Placental site trophoblastic tumour	
	Epithelioid trophoblastic tumour	

Molar pregnancy

Also known as *hydatidiform mole (HM)*, a molar pregnancy results when there is over-growth of fetal chorionic tissue in the uterus (Wang et al 2017). They can be partial or complete, and women usually present with bleeding, enlarged uterus and excessive vomiting. Diagnosis is with ultrasound scan, and treatment is conservative, with evacuation of the uterus under general anaesthetic, with only about 8% requiring chemotherapy (Seekl et al 2010). As these tumours secrete human chorionic gonadotrophin (hCG), the success of their removal and treatment can be monitored by serial serum and urine hCG levels (Nwabuobii et al 2017). Prognosis and further treatment regimens are informed by FIGO (International Federation of Gynaecology and Obstetrics) staging (FIGO 2002).

Gestational trophoblastic neoplasia

This malignant cancer develops when, despite surgical removal of a molar pregnancy, the disease persists, as indicated when hCG levels remain elevated. As this cancer can become metastatic and therefore lethal, a programme of chemotherapy is indicated, with a high success rate (Taylor et al 2013).

REFLECTION ON THE TRIGGER SCENARIO

Look back on the trigger scenario.

Claire came out of the shower with her heart pounding. She quickly dried herself and went and sat on her bed. She gingerly ran her fingers over the spot on her left breast where she thought she had felt a lump. There was no doubt – there it was. She fumbled for her phone and with hands shaking, rang her mum who said, 'Are you sure, love? You know your boobs do change when you are pregnant.'

We have seen (see Table 2.3) how some symptoms could be perceived as pregnancy related rather than a possible cancer sign. The scenario is one that highlights the potential for signs of cancer to be brushed aside and considered a normal part of pregnancy. Now that you are familiar with some of the issues women face when they experience cancer during pregnancy, you should have insight into how the scenario relates to the evidence. The jigsaw model will now be used to explore the trigger scenario in more depth.

Effective communication

Claire has identified a health concern that she needs to discuss with a health professional. Being able to do this in a timely manner is key when cancer is suspected. We know that women often turn to their family and friends at times when they want advice or reassurance. Questions that arise from the scenario might include: Does Claire know how to contact her midwife about the discovery of a lump in her breast? Does Claire have access to a direct point of contact for urgent issues? How might Claire's midwife respond to her concerns? Where would the conversation be documented? How would the midwife escalate Claire's discovery of a breast lump? How would she follow up what further action was taken following referral?

Woman-centred care

If cancer is diagnosed, it is important that Claire receives care that meets her unique needs for both emotional and clinical care. Claire's named midwife is well placed to ensure that care takes account of her particular hopes and fears for the pregnancy. Questions that arise from the scenario might include: How can Claire's midwife help her to focus on her developing baby and becoming a mother? How will Claire accommodate the role of patient throughout her treatment? How will Claire be involved in decisions about her treatment during pregnancy? How can the midwife ensure that Claire is involved in decisions about her birthing options whilst maintaining a safe environment for her?

Using best evidence

Treatment options for cancer are constantly evolving. Midwives will not routinely care for women who are diagnosed with cancer during pregnancy. Questions that arise from the scenario might include: How can midwives keep up to date with new technologies and advances in detection, diagnosis and treatment of rare conditions? What are the 'gold standard' sources of evidence? What is the role of cancer charities in providing a platform for summarizing evidence? Should Claire be involved in clinical trials regarding treatment options during pregnancy?

Professional and legal issues

Midwives have a duty to provide safe and effective care to women in their care. They must maintain confidentiality and respect the woman's wishes even when they decline treatment that may be life-saving. Questions that arise from the scenario might include: How would you respond if a woman in your care declined cancer treatment during her pregnancy? What would your legal and professional actions be in that instance? Who would you go to for support and guidance if you felt upset or traumatized by a clinical situation? How would you support a colleague who was having difficulties accepting a woman's decision to decline treatment?

Team working

When cancer is suspected or diagnosed, it is essential that the woman receives care from the most appropriate health professional. Referral to specialist services is key to ensure that the woman receives counselling regarding her treatment options. However, the woman is still an expectant parent and needs to engage with the obstetric and midwifery team to receive coordinated maternity care.

Questions that arise from the scenario might include: Which specialist would need to be involved in a coordinated programme of oncological and obstetric care? Who will be the lead carer throughout the pregnancy? How will members of the team communicate with each other?

Clinical dexterity

Women who are diagnosed with cancer during pregnancy may be advised to have surgery to remove the tumour. Diagnosis may also have involved invasive interventions such as biopsy. It is likely that the midwife will be called to assess the woman's progress during her treatment and will therefore potentially encounter wound sites, drains and the need to undertake clinical observations. Questions that arise from the scenario might include: How will Claire's midwife develop her knowledge and skills around postoperative care? Are these skills transferable? Who else might be available for advice regarding postoperative care and support? What wound closure methods are practised following mastectomy? When and how are they removed?

Models of care

We have seen how important multi-professional care will be for women with a cancer diagnosis during pregnancy. This may limit her choice for a midwifery-led approach to labour and birth, which she may have been hoping for. However, the midwife can provide a real anchor of support for Claire as she negotiates this complex journey of testing, diagnosis and treatment. Questions that arise from the scenario might include: What models of care exist where you work to support women with complex medical or social needs? Are there options for continuity of midwife care throughout the antenatal, intrapartum and postnatal periods? What opportunities are there for pregnant women to get to know other women in their local community?

Safe environment

Cancer care in pregnancy is complex and multi-faceted. There are many considerations to take into account, for example, drug regimens, fetal growth and wellbeing in combination with cancer monitoring and the impact of treatments. Questions that arise from the scenario might include: What strategies are in place to ensure that Claire receives a timely response to any physical or emotional concerns? Are Claire's medical and obstetric notes available to all members of the team? Does Claire know how to monitor her own health and wellbeing and when to seek medical advice and attention? How does continuity of carer contribute to safer maternity care?

Promotes health

In this scenario Claire's mother is inclined to consider a pregnancy reason for her daughter's breast lump. This is understandable given the rarity of discovering a cancer at this time. However, this is an opportunity to encourage and extol the importance of breast screening and self-examination throughout the life cycle. A cancer diagnosis also has the potential to interfere with a woman's desire to offer her baby the best start in life, such as a vaginal birth at term and establishing breastfeeding. Questions that arise from the scenario might include: What opportunities are there to engage the wider family in public health initiatives to promote health? What additional professional/third-sector groups might Claire engage with to support her physical and emotional wellbeing? What systems are in place where you work to offer donor breastmilk to babies of women whose drug therapy precludes breastfeeding?

Further scenarios

The following scenarios enable you to consider how specific situations influence the care the midwife provides. Use the jigsaw model to explore the issues raised in the scenario.

SCENARIO 1

Carol had a history of long-standing mental illness. She had persistent vomiting throughout her pregnancy and was prescribed anti-emetics but with no effect. She was referred to the ear, nose and throat (ENT) department at her local hospital, as her GP suspected labyrinthitis, but no ENT cause for her symptoms was found. She was also experiencing severe headaches and eventually collapsed. A subsequent neurological examination then revealed raised intracranial pressure secondary to a brain tumour.

Practice point

This is a summary based on a case presented in the Confidential Enquiry into Maternal Deaths (Knight et al 2015:57), which focuses on care of women who died following malignancy. Whilst the narrative acknowledges that earlier diagnosis may not have changed the outcome, it highlights the danger of health professionals working in 'silos' and not thinking outside of their own speciality and taking a wider view. It leads to the recommendation that all women with new-onset headaches should have a neurological examination (Knight et al 2015:58).

Questions that could be asked are:
1. Did the woman's history of mental health problems cloud the significance of her physical symptoms?
2. Is there a role for the midwife to consider non-obstetric causes of her symptoms?
3. What was her vomiting caused by?
4. What are the elements of the neurological examination (see Chapter 9)?
5. Who else could have been involved in her care?
6. How might an earlier diagnosis of brain tumour have impacted on her pregnancy care?

SCENARIO 2

Hannah was 8 weeks pregnant with her first baby and attended her booking appointment with her midwife, Sally. During the conversation Sally asked Hannah when she had her last cervical smear. Hannah looked down and paused, then replied, 'I haven't had one yet...I kept meaning to, but I'm too scared. My friend told me that it hurts'.

The cervical screening programme is available to all women aged over 25 years in the UK and includes testing for HPV. Eligible women are invited by letter to attend their local GP clinic, where a practice nurse trained in the procedure can take the smear. There are a range of reasons why not all women take up this offer, from fear of pain, not understanding the importance, embarrassment or simply because they work shifts which make access difficult.

Questions that could be asked are:
1. What is the national uptake of cervical screening?
2. What is the incidence of a positive screening result?
3. What should Sally advise Hannah to do?
4. What information is available to Hannah to help her make an informed choice?
5. How can Sally promote the uptake of this important screening test?
6. Can a smear be taken in pregnancy?

Conclusion

The midwife is the lynch pin for women who are receiving care from the multi-professional team, as she can provide continuity and consistency throughout the pathway. The role of the midwife caring for a woman with cancer in her childbearing years is to ensure she is still treated like a mother, with compassion, kindness and hope.

Resources

Andersson, T.M., Johansson, A.L., Fredriksson, I., Lambe, M., 2015. Cancer during pregnancy and the postpartum period: a population-based study. Cancer 121, 2072–2077.

Cancer Research UK https://www.cancerresearchuk.org/

Breast cancer care https://www.breastcancercare.org.uk/

Fertility preservation. Breast Cancer Care. Patient video stories https://www.breastcancercare.org.uk/information-support/facing-breast-cancer/breast-cancer-in-younger-women/fertility-pregnancy-breast-cancer-treatment/preserving-fertility

Jo's cervical cancer trust https://www.jostrust.org.uk/get-involved/campaign/time-test

Leukaemia Care (Blood cancer Charity) https://www.leukaemiacare.org.uk/support-and-information/information-about-blood-cancer/blood-cancer-information/

Macmillan Cancer Support https://www.macmillan.org.uk

Mummy's Star. UK and Ireland Charity Supporting pregnancy through cancer and beyond. Also offers support to health professionals caring for women with cancer. http://www.mummysstar.org/

PREDICT website for assisting women make informed decisions about breast cancer treatments http://www.predict.nhs.uk/index.html

References

Alexander, A., Samlowski, W., Grossman, D., et al., 2003. Metastatic melanoma in pregnancy: risk of transplacental metastases in the infant. J. Clin. Oncol. 21 (11), 2179–2186.

Ali, S., Jones, G., Culligan, D., et al., 2015. Guidelines for the diagnosis and management of acute myeloid leukaemia in pregnancy. Br. J. Haematol. 170 (4), 487–495.

Amant, F., Deckers, S., Van Calsteren, K., et al., 2010. Breast cancer in pregnancy: recommendations of an international consensus meeting. Eur. J. Cancer 46, 3158–3168.

Amant, F., Loibl, S., Neven, P., Van Calsteren, K., 2012. Breast cancer in pregnancy. Lancet 379 (9815), 570–579.

Amant, F., Vandenbroucke, T., Verheecke, M., et al., 2015. Pediatric outcome after maternal cancer diagnosed during pregnancy. N. Engl. J. Med. 373 (19), 1824–1834.

Bachanova, V.M., Connors, J., 2013. Hodgkin lymphoma in pregnancy. Curr. Hematol. Malig. Rep. 8 (3), 1–7.

Bradford, P.T., Anderson, W.F., Purdue, M.P., et al., 2010. Rising melanoma incidence rates of the trunk among younger women in the United States Cancer Epidemiol. Biomark. Prev. 19, 2401–2406.

Cancer Centre, 2018. Hodgkin lymphoma symptoms. Available from: https://www.cancercenter.com/hodgkin-lymphoma/symptoms/.

Cancer Research UK, 2017. Breast MRI scan. Available from: https://www.cancerresearchuk.org/about-cancer/breast-cancer/getting-diagnosed/tests-diagnose/breast-mri-scan.

Cancer research UK. Cervical cancer survival. Available from: https://www.cancerresearchuk.org/health-professional/cancer-statistics/statistics-by-cancer-type/cervical-cancer#heading-Three.

Candido Dos Reis, F., Wishart, G., Dicks, E., et al., 2017. An updated PREDICT breast cancer prognostication and treatment benefit prediction model with independent validation. Breast Cancer Res. 19 (1), 58.

Castanon, A., Lundy, R., Brocklehurst, P., et al., 2014. Risk of preterm delivery with increasing depth of excision for cervical intraepithelial neoplasia in England: nested case control study. BMJ 349 (7982), 12.

Chelghoum, Y., Vey, N., Raffoux, E., et al., 2005. Acute leukemia during pregnancy – A report on 37 patients and a review of the literature. Cancer 104 (1), 110–117.

Davison, J., Narain, S., Mcewan, A., 2017. Cancer in pregnancy. Obstet. Gynaecol. Reprod. Med. 27 (8), 251–255.

FIGO, 2002. Oncology Committee Report FIGO staging for gestational trophoblastic neoplasia 2000. FIGO Oncology Committee. Int. J. Gynecol. Obstet. 77, 285–287.

George-Carey, R., Koniman, W., ParisaeiHodgkin, M., 2017. Hodgkin's lymphoma and pregnancy. BJOG 124 (S1), 167–168.

Hermandez, E., 2018. Gestational trophoblastic Neoplasia. Medscape https://emedicine.medscape.com/article/279116-overview.

International Commission on Radiological Protection, 2003. Biological effects after prenatal irradiation (embryo and fetus). Ann. ICRP 33, 205–206.

Kal, H., Struikmans, H., 2005. Radiotherapy during pregnancy: fact and fiction. Lancet Oncol. 6 (5), 328–333.

Karen, B., Lewing, M., Alan, S., Gamis, M., 2010. Lymphoma. In: Holcomb, G. (Ed.), Ashcraft's Pediatric Surgery, Fifth ed. Elsevier, Edinburgh.

Kent, E., Gorman, M., Orme-Evans, K., Caughey, A., 2015. Morbidity and mortality associated with breast cancer diagnosis in pregnancy: a retrospective cohort study. Am. J. Obstet. Gynecol. 212 (1), S383.

Knight, M., Nair, M., Tuffnell, D., et al. (Eds.) on behalf of MBRRACE-UK, 2017. Saving Lives, Improving Mothers' Care – Lessons learned to inform maternity care from the UK and Ireland Confidential Enquiries into Maternal Deaths and Morbidity 2013–15. Oxford: National Perinatal Epidemiology Unit, University of Oxford. Available from: https://www.npeu.ox.ac.uk/downloads/files/mbrrace-uk/reports/MBRRACE-UK%20Maternal%20Report%20 2017%20-%20Web.pdf.

Knight, M., Tuffnell, D., Kenyon, S., et al. (Eds.) on behalf of MBRRACE-UK, 2015. Saving Lives, Improving Mothers' Care – Surveillance of maternal deaths in the UK 2011-13 and lessons learned to inform maternity care from the UK and Ireland Confidential Enquiries into Maternal Deaths and Morbidity 2009-13. Oxford: National Perinatal Epidemiology Unit, University of Oxford. Available from: https://www.npeu.ox.ac.uk/downloads/files/mbrrace-uk/reports/MBRRACE-UK%20Maternal%20Report%202015.pdf.

Ksheerasagar, S., Monnappa, G., Venkatesh, N., 2017. Breast cancer in pregnancy. J. Obstet. Gynecol. India 67 (6), 442–444.

Kyrgiou, M., Mitra, A., Arbyn, M., et al., 2015. Fertility and early pregnancy outcomes after conservative treatment for cervical intraepithelial neoplasia. Cochrane Database Syst. Rev. (9), CD008478, doi:10.1002/14651858.CD008478.pub2.

Monteiro, D., Trajano, A., Menezes, D., et al., 2013. Breast cancer during pregnancy and chemotherapy: a systematic review. Rev. Assoc. Med. Bras. 59 (2), 174–180.

Münter, M., Wengenroth, M., Fehrenbacher, G., et al., 2010. Heavy ion radiotherapy during pregnancy. Fertil. Steril. 94 (6), 2329.e5–2329.e7.

Navrozoglou, I., Vrekousis, T., Kontostolis, E., et al., 2008. Breast cancer during pregnancy: a mini-review. Eur. J. Surg. Oncol. 34, 837–843.

NHS England, 2017. Don't let embarrassment prevent cervical cancer screening. Available from: https://www.england.nhs.uk/south/2017/01/20/cervical-cancer-prevention/.

NICE, 2009, revised 2018. Early and locally advanced breast cancer: diagnosis and management. NICE Guideline 101. Available from: https://www.nice.org.uk/guidance/ng101/chapter/Recommendations.

NICE, 2017. Clinical Knowledge Summaries for cervical cancer. Cervical cancer and HPV. Available from: https://cks.nice.org.uk/cervical-cancer-and-hpv#!scenario:1.

Nitsche, S., Braunstein, G., 2017. Chapter 21 endocrine changes in pregnancy. In: Melmed, S., Polonsky, K. (Eds.), Williams Textbook of Endocrinology, 13th ed. Elsevier, Edinburgh.

Nwabuobii, C., Arlier, S., Schatz, F., et al., 2017. 2017 HCG: biological functions and clinical applications. Int. J. Mol. Sci. 18 (10), 2037.

Patenaude, Y., Pugash, D., Lim, K., et al., 2014. The use of magnetic resonance imaging in the obstetric patient. J. Obstet. Gynaecol. Can. 36, 349–363.

Pokhrel, S., Quigley, M., Fox-Rushby, J., 2015. Potential economic impacts from improving breastfeeding rates in the UK. Arch. Dis. Child. 100 (4), 334–340. doi:10.1136/archdischild-2014-306701.

Public Health England, 2018. Stoptober. Available from: https://campaignre-sources.phe.gov.uk/resources/campaigns/6-stoptober/overview.

Renfrew, M., Pokhrel, S., Quigley, M., 2012. Preventing disease and saving resources: the potential contribution of increasing breastfeeding rates in the UK. UNICEF.

Royal College of Obstetricians and Gynaecologists, 2015. Green-top Guideline 37a: Reducing the Risk of Venous Thromboembolism During Pregnancy and the Puerperium. Available from: https://www.rcog.org.uk/globalassets/documents/guidelines/gtg-37a.pdf. (Accessed 31 July 2015).

Samarasinghe, A., Shafi, M., 2014. Cancer in pregnancy. Obstet. Gynaecol. Reprod. Med. 24 (11), 333–339.

Seckl, M., Sebire, N., Berkowitz, R., 2010. Gestational trophoblastic disease. Lancet 376 (9742), 717–729.

Taylor, F., Grew, T., Everard, J., et al., 2013. The outcome of patients with low risk gestational trophoblastic neoplasia treated with single agent intramuscular methotrexate and oral folinic acid. Eur. J. Cancer 49 (15), 3184–3190.

Todd, S., Driscoll, M., 2017. Prognosis for women diagnosed with melanoma during, before, or after pregnancy: weighing the evidence. Int. J. Womens Dermatol. 3 (1), 26–29.

Tombola group, 2009. Biopsy and selective recall compared with immediate large loop excision in management of women with low grade abnormal cervical cytology referred for colposcopy: multicentre randomised controlled trial. BMJ 339 (2), B2548.

Walker, J., Wang, A., Kroumpouzos, G., Weinstock, M., 2016. Cutaneous tumors in pregnancy. Clin. Dermatol. 34 (3), 359–367.

Wang, Q., Fu, J., Hu, L., et al., 2017. Prophylactic chemotherapy for hydatidiform mole to prevent gestational trophoblastic neoplasia. Cochrane Database Syst. Rev. (9), Art. No.: CD007289, doi:10.1002/14651858.CD007289.pub3.

Zhang, X., Gao, Y., Yang, Y., 2015. Treatment and prognosis of cervical cancer associated with pregnancy: analysis of 20 cases from a Chinese tumor institution. J. Zhejiang Univ. Sci. B 16 (5), 388–394.

CHAPTER 3

Hypertensive disorders in pregnancy

TRIGGER SCENARIO

Olivia is 42 years old and following her second cycle of in vitro fertiliza-tion (IVF). She discovers that she is pregnant for the first time. Whilst she is overjoyed, she is also concerned that as an older pregnant woman, she and her baby have a greater chance of complications such as hyper-tension. Her blood pressure is borderline, and with a family history of hypertension, she has read a lot about these potential risk factors. Olivia wants to be as involved as possible in decision-making about the care and management of her pregnancy.

Introduction

Hypertension refers to persistent high blood pressure. It is associated with conditions such as diabetes and obesity; it may be symptomless, and in the UK as many as 7 million people are living with cardiovascular disorders such as coronary heart disease, vascular dementia and stroke (British Heart Foundation (BHF) 2018). Hypertensive disorders in childbearing women are associated with maternal and fetal or neonatal morbidity and mortality (Harding et al 2016; Traquilli et al 2014) and pose specific challenges for the women, their families and those providing their maternity care. This chapter provides a brief review of the phys-iology relating to cardiovascular changes in pregnancy and the signifi-cance of hypertension for the mother and baby. It summarizes the main types of hypertensive disorders in pregnancy and identifies the women at increased risk of developing these. Essential aspects of multi-professional and midwifery care are discussed, and consideration is given to the phys-ical and psychosocial impact of hypertensive disorders in pregnancy for the women affected.

Physiological changes to circulation in pregnancy

Blood pressure (BP) reflects the relationship between cardiac output and the resistance of the peripheral blood vessels; it varies according to health, activity and emotion, and is regulated through integrated hormonal and neurological controls (Cowan et al 2017). During pregnancy, the following physiological adaptations occur:

+ Blood volume and cardiac output increase.
+ Peripheral vascular resistance decreases.

The endothelium (lining of the blood vessels) plays an important role in controlling the mother's cardiovascular functioning, and increased fluid transfer across the endothelium can predispose pregnant women to oedema.

BP usually remains relatively stable during pregnancy, although a slight fall of 5 to 10 mm Hg may occur during the second trimester when the decrease in peripheral resistance is greater than the increase in blood volume and cardiac output. There may be an increase in BP during labour when uterine contractions force increased amounts of blood from the uterine body into the general circulation (McCarthy & Kenny 2010).

Hypertension in pregnancy

The underlying cause of hypertension in pregnancy is uncertain but is thought to result from a combination of factors. Hypertension in pregnancy may be associated with atypical endothelium and abnormalities in blood clotting factors and blood flow, which predispose women to increased blood clotting (McCarthy & Kenny 2010). Hypertensive disorders affect 3% to 10% of pregnancies (Hutcheon et al 2011; Ukah et al 2018), comprising approximately 1% chronic hypertension, 5% to 6% gestational hypertension and 1% to 2% pre-eclampsia (Magee et al 2014). Hypertensive disorders are a leading cause in maternal, fetal and neonatal mortality and morbidity. Over recent decades in the UK, the number of childbearing women with hypertensive disorders who have died from conditions such as intracranial haemorrhage, eclampsia and cerebral oedema, pulmonary oedema, coagulation disorders and liver failure or rupture has decreased significantly, and the incidence of eclampsia almost halved between 1992 and 2007. Nevertheless, improvements in care might have avoided 13 of the 14 maternal deaths relating to hypertension during 2009–2014 (Harding et al 2016). Women with pre-eclampsia are more likely to need admission to an intensive care unit and have an increased chance of placental abruption (Hutcheon et al 2011). Maternal hypertensive disorders also impact on the fetus and neonate; in the 2017 Confidential Enquiry into Perinatal Mortality, Heazell and Evans (2017) reported that 7% of women whose baby was stillborn had hypertensive disorders. Fetal growth restriction is also a consequence of maternal hypertension along with iatrogenic preterm birth, neonatal death, respiratory complications and cerebral palsy (Hutcheon et al 2011; Mol et al 2016).

Which women are affected by hypertension in pregnancy?

Whilst maternal risk factors and individual tests do not predict adverse maternal outcomes (Traquilli et al 2014; Ukah et al 2018), certain groups of women are identified as being at greater risk (Table 3.1). For instance, women with twin pregnancies are two to three times more likely to develop pre-eclampsia than women with singleton pregnancies, although they may not experience correspondingly higher levels of hypertensive-related maternal or fetal mortality and morbidity (Connolly et al 2016), and Ferrazzani et al (2015:176) suggest there may be a 'beneficial role of uncomplicated hypertension in twin pregnancies.'

Pre-existing diabetes is associated with pre-eclampsia if women's glycaemic control is poor prior to 20 weeks' gestation, as well as if they have renal damage and are nulliparous (Kourtis 2012). Risk factors alone might identify around 30% of women who develop pre-eclampsia (Mol et al 2016). Consideration of multiple factors can further aid identification of women who are at high risk (Ukah et al 2018).

Table 3.1: **Risk factors for pre-eclampsia**

High-risk factors for pre-eclampsia:
- Hypertensive disorder in previous pregnancy
- Chronic hypertension
- Chronic kidney disease
- Immune disorder, e.g. antiphospholipid syndrome
- Type 1 or type 2 diabetes

Moderate-risk factors for pre-eclampsia:
- Nulliparous
- Primipaternity (new partner or pregnancy interval ≥5 years)*
- Short relationship with father (≤6 months) before the pregnancy*
- ≥40 years old
- ≥10 years since previous pregnancy
- Booking body mass index (BMI) ≥35 kg/m²
- Pre-eclampsia in family history
- Multiple pregnancy
- African American ethnic origin*

*Additional risk factors as identified by Traquilli et al (2014) and not included in NICE (2010) recommendation for prophylactic low-dose aspirin.
From (NICE 2010; Traquilli et al 2014)

Significant pregnancy-related hypertensive disorders

There are different classifications of hypertensive disorders in pregnancy (Table 3.2), and the severity of hypertension varies from mild to severe (Table 3.3) (National Institute for Health and Care Excellence (NICE) 2010).

Chronic hypertension

This condition has no identifiable cause in most cases (essential hypertension). In around 10% of cases this is secondary to underlying disease, such as renal, vascular, connective tissue or endocrine disorders (Heazell et al 2010; Ryan & McCarthy 2018). Chronic hypertension

Table 3.2: **Classification of hypertensive disorders in pregnancy**

Condition	Definition
Chronic hypertension	Hypertension presenting prior to 20 weeks' gestation; women may already be taking anti-hypertensive medication
Gestational hypertension	New hypertension occurring after 20 weeks' gestation; no significant proteinuria; women have an increased chance of pre-eclampsia and hypertension in later life
Pre-eclampsia	New hypertension occurring after 20 weeks' gestation; significant proteinuria (≥300 mg protein in 24 hours; spot test protein-creatinine ratio (PCR) 30)
Severe pre-eclampsia	Pre-eclampsia with severe hypertension, with or without symptoms and/or biochemical and/or haematological changes
Eclampsia	Convulsions associated with pre-eclampsia
HELLP syndrome	Haemolysis, elevated liver enzymes, low platelets

From (NICE 2010)

Table 3.3: **Severity of hypertension in pregnancy**

Classification	Range
Mild hypertension	Diastolic 90–99 Systolic 140–149
Moderate hypertension	Diastolic 100–109 Systolic 150–159
Severe hypertension	Diastolic 110+ Systolic 160+

From (NICE 2010)

increased a woman's potential for adverse pregnancy outcomes and can be super-imposed by pre-eclampsia (Magee et al 2014). For women with chronic hypertension, pre-conception care can be advantageous (Bramham et al 2014), incorporating a review of anti-hypertensive medications, since some of these (such as angiotensin-converting enzyme (ACE) inhibitors) are associated with congenital abnormalities (McCarthy & Kenny 2015; NICE 2010). Women with underlying renal disease are particularly at risk of adverse outcomes (Heazell et al 2010), and some hypertensive conditions – for instance, pulmonary hypertension – are believed to pose such a significant threat to maternal health that women may be advised to avoid pregnancy (Pieper & Hoendermis 2011). Investigations in early pregnancy can aid the diagnosis and management of these underlying conditions.

Gestational hypertension

This form of hypertension occurs initially after 20 weeks' gestation and typically resolves by 12 weeks following the birth (Hutcheon et al 2011). Early onset (<32 to 34 weeks' gestation) is associated with greater risk of adversity and the development of pre-eclampsia in 25% to 35% of cases (Magee et al 2014; Traquilli et al 2014).

Pre-eclampsia

This much-feared disease process traditionally presents with hypertension and proteinuria. However, recent definitions, which include end-organ disorders such as renal insufficiency, liver damage, neurological or haematological problems, uteroplacental dysfunction and intrauterine growth restriction (Mol et al 2016; Traquilli et al 2014), suggest that proteinuria is not *essential* for a diagnosis of pre-eclampsia. Traquilli et al (2014:98) recommend that 'all asymptomatic women with less than severe hypertension (140-159/90-109) and no dipstick proteinuria' should have biochemical tests to exclude maternal organ dysfunction and consequently exclude pre-eclampsia. Furthermore, whilst the progress and outcomes of pre-eclampsia may differ between women, the International Society for the Study of Hypertension in Pregnancy (ISSHP) (Traquilli et al 2014) warn against mild/moderate/severe classifications, since the course of pre-eclampsia can deteriorate suddenly, leading to major maternal and perinatal adversity. All women with pre-eclampsia should therefore be cared for based on this understanding. Early-onset pre-eclampsia (before 32 to 34 weeks' gestation) is associated with particular severity and poorer outcomes and may be associated with underlying environmental or genetic factors which affect placentation (Hutcheon et al 2011).

Eclampsia

An eclamptic seizure may be the first sign of a pregnancy-related hypertensive condition (Repke & Norwitz 2010). Seizures are usually self-limiting but are associated with poor maternal and fetal outcomes such as coma, intracranial haemorrhage, respiratory distress and perinatal death (Hutcheon et al 2011). Declining eclampsia rates in developed countries are attributed to better antenatal care, planned early birth for women with pre-eclampsia and the use of magnesium sulphate (Hutcheon et al 2011). Expectant management is contraindicated for women with eclampsia, and once their condition is stabilized, plans should be made for birth (Repke & Norwitz 2010). If a woman does not recover following a seizure or has focal neurological symptoms, neuroimaging should be performed urgently and neurological specialists involved in their care (Harding et al 2016).

> ## Activity
> What is HELLP syndrome?
> How is it related to pre-eclampsia, and how is it managed?

Team approach to care and management

Women who present with hypertensive disorders in pregnancy should be referred for an appraisal of their condition by a senior obstetrician so that an ongoing plan of care can be developed and shared (NICE 2010). The plan should be regularly reviewed and amended accordingly, with input from a multi-disciplinary team (Harding et al 2016), which may involve hypertensive (NICE 2010), high-risk pregnancy, anaesthetic, haematology and other appropriate specialists. Depending on the severity of their condition and local provision of services, women's care may involve hospital admission or day care.

Assessments and investigations

Establishing the diagnosis and progression of hypertensive disorders relies on multiple sources of information about maternal and fetal wellbeing. Assessments may need to be repeated according to the clinical picture so that management can be discussed, implemented and evaluated (Magee et al 2014; NICE 2010). Investigations can aid in providing differential diagnoses and detecting organ dysfunction or adverse outcomes and the seriousness of these (Magee et al 2014). Midwives can help women understand the practical aspects and significance of these investigations.

Women with pre-eclampsia can be asymptomatic; therefore careful midwifery assessment can aid in the diagnosis. This begins at the first midwifery appointment when a woman's booking history or physical assessment may reveal risk factors. Where these or other deviations from normal are identified, midwives have a responsibility to refer women to the most appropriate health professional (Nursing and Midwifery Council 2015) and to ensure that women understand the reasons for referral to a consultant obstetrician.

Clinical observations

BP should be measured and urine tested for protein at every antepartum contact with women – the frequency of this will be determined by the woman's condition (NICE 2010). Measuring BP must be accurate and consistent: for detailed guidance about how to measure BP and perform urinalysis accurately, see Baston and Hall (2017) *Midwifery Essentials: Basics*.

The identification of proteinuria contributes to a diagnosis of infection, renal disease in early pregnancy and pre-eclampsia after 20 weeks' gestation (Magee et al 2014). Urinalysis should ideally be performed using either an automated reagent strip reader or spot urinary protein-creatinine ratio (PCR) in the hospital setting. Readings of 1+ protein on dipstick indicate further investigation, and significant proteinuria is diagnosed as urinary PCR >30 mg/mmol or 300 mg protein in a 24-hour urine collection (NICE 2010).

Significant proteinuria is central to anticipating outcomes for both mother and baby (McCarthy & Kenny 2015), although the degree of proteinuria is not indicative of complications such as placental abruption or HELLP syndrome (Mol et al 2016). If PCR >230 mg/mmol, this suggests that nephrotic-range proteinuria has been reached and prophylaxis against thromboembolism is required (Traquilli et al 2014).

Enabling women to identify signs and symptoms of pre-eclampsia can avoid delays in diagnosis and management. Women should be advised that if they develop severe headache; blurred vision; severe upper abdominal pain; vomiting; or sudden facial, hand or foot oedema, they should seek immediate advice from a midwife or doctor (NICE 2010).

Activity

Access the Action on Pre-Eclampsia (APEC) website and the learning resources available for health professionals. Compare the information written for professionals with information provided for parents. This might help you explain complex aspects of hypertensive disorders using woman-centred language.

Biochemical testing

All pregnant women with hypertensive disorders should be offered routine antenatal blood tests. In addition, whilst some of the following biochemical investigations may have limited value in predicting complications (Mol et al 2016), they, too, form part of the overall understanding of the woman's condition:

+ **Kidney function:** Urea and electrolytes; creatinine may be increased due to haemoconcentration and/or renal damage; albumin may be decreased in response to the acute illness, renal damage or crystalloid infusion (Magee et al 2014).
+ **Full blood count:** May demonstrate haemoconcentration due to intravascular fluid depletion or low haemoglobin levels due to haemolysis (Magee et al 2014); may reveal thrombocytopaenia and reduced platelets associated with HELLP syndrome (McCarthy & Kenny 2015); coagulation screening is indicated if the platelet count is below 100×10^9 platelets/L blood (Mol et al 2016).
+ **Liver function** (such as transaminases and bilirubin): Help to exclude HELLP syndrome (McCarthy & Kenny 2015); aspartate transaminase (AST) and alanine transaminase (ALT) levels are gestation related and increase with liver damage (Cowan et al 2017).

It is important to remember that although positive results contribute to a diagnosis of pre-eclampsia, negative results do not exclude it (Cowan et al 2017).

Assessing fetal wellbeing

Poor placental perfusion associated with pre-eclampsia is linked with intrauterine growth restriction and oligohydramnios. Babies born to mothers with pre-eclampsia may have a birth weight that is 5% less than babies born to unaffected mothers; this increases to a difference of up to 23% when mothers have early-onset pre-eclampsia (Bokslag et al 2016). Assessing and plotting fetal growth on a customized chart and asking women to observe and report any concerns regarding fetal activity can therefore contribute to the overall assessment (Traquilli et al 2014).

Ultrasound measurements of fetal growth, amniotic fluid index and umbilical artery Doppler velocimetry contribute to an understanding of fetal wellbeing and management choices (McCarthy & Kenny 2015). Fetal growth restriction associated with pre-eclampsia may be asymmetrical or, in early or severe cases, symmetrical (Magee et al 2014). Umbilical artery Doppler ultrasonography may be useful in predicting pre-eclampsia, particularly when this is combined with identification of risk factors and maternal serum biomarkers such as placental protein-13 (PP-13) and pregnancy-associated plasma protein-A (PAPP-A) (McLeod 2008). Abnormalities in umbilical artery Doppler readings, such as increased resistance and absent or reverse end-diastolic flow, are not specific to the *cause* of placental dysfunction, but features such as unilateral or bilateral notching and increased pulsatility index can support a diagnosis of placental insufficiency, including that resulting from pre-eclampsia (Magee et al 2014). Furthermore, oligohydramnios and abnormalities in umbilical artery Doppler measurements can be useful in predicting the risk of stillbirth, and incorporating these results with other assessments is recommended in planning care (Magee et al 2014).

Abnormalities in fetal heart traces such as decreased variability may present with pre-eclampsia (Magee et al 2014), and midwives have a responsibility to recognize the importance of timely fetal heart monitoring, deviations from normal and appropriate escalation in response to changes.

Management
Prophylaxis

There is no universal prevention against pre-eclampsia, although aspirin and calcium appear to offer some benefits (Traquilli et al 2014). The CLASP Collaborative Group (CCG) (1994) found that women who take low-dose aspirin from early pregnancy are less likely to develop early-onset pre-eclampsia. Pre-eclampsia has a range of manifestations, and low-dose aspirin may not be helpful for all women. Women at high risk of early-onset pre-eclampsia may benefit most, although accurately identifying these women is difficult. Pre-eclampsia can begin from 20 weeks' gestation (CCG 1994); therefore the benefits are greatest when prophylaxis is commenced prior to 16 weeks' gestation (Bujold et al 2010; Magee et al 2014). NICE (2010) recommends that women with one high-risk factor or more than one moderate-risk factor (see Table 3.1) are offered prophylactic low-dose (75 mg/day) aspirin from 12 weeks' gestation to the birth of their baby.

Activity

What are the potential risks of taking low-dose aspirin for the mother and/or her baby?

Calcium supplements of 1 g/day or more can reduce the risk of pre-eclampsia for women who have a low calcium intake (Magee et al 2014; Mol et al 2016; Traquilli et al 2014), and although folic acid supplementation is not recommended solely for reducing the risk of hypertensive disorders in pregnancy (NICE 2010), continued use throughout pregnancy may contribute to avoiding gestational hypertension and pre-eclampsia (De Ocampo et al 2018).

Anti-hypertensive medication

Anti-hypertensive drugs do not prevent pre-eclampsia but can halve the risk of severe hypertension (Bramham et al 2014; Magee et al 2014). Maintaining BP readings below 150/100 is essential to avoid complications such as intracranial haemorrhage (Harding et al 2016); this can be particularly important for women who require a general anaesthetic, since induction of anaesthesia can cause a surge in BP. Target BP levels may be lower (140/90) for women with conditions such as kidney disease (NICE 2010). The primary anti-hypertensive drug of choice in the UK is labetalol, although methyldopa and nifedipine are recommended alternatives (NICE 2010).

Labetalol is a combined β-adrenoceptor and α-adrenoceptor blocker which controls BP quickly. If there is no response to oral medication or this is contraindicated, labetalol can be administered by intravenous infusion. It is contraindicated in women with asthma and should be used cautiously for women with cardiac disease (McCarthy & Kenny 2015; Ryan & McCarthy 2018) and poorly or tightly controlled diabetes (Daskas et al 2013). There have been concerns that maternal labetalol use is linked with neonatal hypoglycaemia. However, these babies may develop hypoglycaemia because of intrauterine growth restriction (Daskas et al 2013) or prematurity (Bokslag et al 2016). By careful observation and facilitating early feeding (where appropriate), midwives and neonatal staff can help avert, detect and manage neonatal hypoglycaemia.

Nifedipine is a calcium channel blocker which is effective for use in pregnancy but has less extensive supporting evidence than labetalol or methyldopa. It can cause severe headaches and should not be administered sublingually during pregnancy, as the rapid fall in BP can reduce placental perfusion, causing fetal hypoxia. The cumulative effect of nifedipine and magnesium sulphate (see later) can cause hypotension; therefore caution and careful monitoring are needed if these are to be administered concurrently (McCarthy & Kenny 2015).

Methyldopa is an α-adrenergic agonist whose use in pregnancy is well recognized. However, methyldopa can have a sedative effect, which can deter women from taking it (McCarthy & Kenny 2015).

Hydralazine is a short-acting anti-hypertensive drug that may be less effective than other drugs and have greater side effects, such as maternal hypotension. Given intravenously, it may be more effective than labetalol.

Anti-convulsant therapy

Magnesium sulphate is the preferred anti-convulsant in the management of pre-eclampsia and can halve the risk of women with pre-eclampsia having a seizure (Traquilli et al 2014). Whilst it can temporarily lower BP following a loading dose, it is not an anti-hypertensive drug (Magee 2014) and, depending on the women's BP, may need to be given in conjunction with anti-hypertensives. In developed countries it is used for women with severe pre-eclampsia and eclampsia to prevent seizures (Mol et al 2016; NICE 2010) and can reduce the associated risk of cerebral palsy in the baby by one-third (Bokslag et al 2016).

Each trust should have guidelines to ensure a consistent approach to the use, monitoring, outcomes and recognition of the side effects of magnesium sulphate (Traquilli et al 2014). The loading dose of magnesium sulphate is 4 g given intravenously over 5 minutes, followed by an intravenous infusion of 1 g per hour for 24 hours after the birth or last seizure (whichever is the latest) (PROMPT Editorial Team 2017). Any recurrent seizures are treated with a further bolus of 2 to 4 g given over 5 minutes (Eclampsia Trial Collaborative Group 1995; Mol et al 2016). Around 97% of magnesium sulphate is excreted in urine (McCarthy & Kenny 2015); therefore oliguria (<100 ml/4 hours) can lead to toxic levels with side effects such as drowsiness, motor paralysis, absent reflexes, respiratory depression and cardiac arrhythmias. A magnesium sulphate infusion should be discontinued in the presence of oliguria, and 10 ml calcium gluconate 10% should be administered by slow intravenous injection as an antidote to toxicity (PROMPT Editorial Team 2017).

Management of an eclamptic seizure

Neurological symptoms such as seizures, altered consciousness, confusion, restlessness or agitation must be managed urgently by senior obstetricians and may indicate intracranial bleeding secondary to hypertension (Harding et al 2016). In the event of a seizure, basic life support measures and control of seizures are the priorities for management (PROMPT Editorial Team 2017), and senior help should be summoned using emergency call systems in the hospital setting or women transferred into hospital using 999 to call an emergency ambulance. During an eclamptic seizure the woman should be protected from injury; airway maintenance and breathing can be managed by placing the woman into a left lateral position and administering high-flow facial oxygen (for further details regarding the management of eclampsia, see Baston and Hall 2018, Vol 6, Chapter 7).

Thromboprophylaxis

Pregnancy increases the risk of women developing venous thromboembolic (VTE) disorders, and these risks are further increased if women are admitted to hospital or develop conditions such as pre-eclampsia (Royal College of Obstetricians and Gynaecologists (RCOG) 2015). Midwives should conduct a VTE assessment at the booking appointment, when there are changes in the woman's condition, on admission to hospital, during labour and again following birth. Depending on the assessment findings, antenatal VTE prophylaxis may be indicated.

Fluid management

Women with pre-eclampsia can retain extravascular fluid, which can lead to pulmonary oedema. Therefore careful fluid management is highly important (Mol et al 2016), with fluid restrictions of around 80 ml/hour in total advocated (1 ml fluid/kg body weight/hour) (PROMPT Editorial Team 2017). This includes avoiding fluid preloading for epidural anaesthetics (Mol et al 2016; NICE 2010). It may be appropriate to adapt fluid management in specific situations, such as women who have haemorrhaged and require fluid replacement; multi-disciplinary management and care are essential.

Accurately measuring and recording all input and output on a fluid chart and calculating a running total will contribute to effective fluid management and reduce the risk of magnesium sulphate toxicity. Monitoring oxygen saturation levels can indicate cardiorespiratory deterioration such as pulmonary oedema or pulmonary embolism (Magee et al 2014), and these observations may be supplemented by central venous pressure monitoring in a high-dependency setting (PROMPT Editorial Team 2017).

Interventions

'The only cure for pre-eclampsia is delivery of the placenta' (Mol et al 2016:1004), and in-patient care for women with severe hypertension or organ dysfunction is strongly and consistently advised (Mol et al 2016; NICE, 2010; Traquilli et al 2014). Bed rest is not advised since this can increase the risk of conditions such as venous thromboembolism and does not prevent pre-eclampsia (Mol et al 2016; NICE 2010).

Timing the birth

Identifying the right time for birth can be a complex decision, based on the balance between maternal morbidity and mortality: escalating hypertension, response to treatment and the risk of ongoing intrauterine growth restriction versus prematurity for the baby (McCarthy & Kenny 2015). However, some of these risks can be mitigated, for example, by the administration of maternal antenatal corticosteroids to accelerate fetal pulmonary development (Bokslag et al 2016). Two doses of bet-amethasone 12 mg 24 hours apart should be offered to women with early-onset pre-eclampsia and considered for women with pre-eclampsia at 35 to 36 weeks' gestation (NICE 2010) or women with gestational hypertension before 34 weeks if birth is likely within 7 days (Magee et al 2014). Midwives need to be aware that following the administration of corticosteroids changes in the fetal heart trace (for instance, relating to variability) may last for about 4 days (Magee et al 2014).

Planning for birth includes the mode of birth, and caesarean section may be advantageous where maternal and fetal conditions are deteriorating quickly (McCarthy & Kenny 2015). Epidural anaesthetic may help prevent further increases in BP and facilitate a 'more controlled second stage' (McCarthy & Kenny 2015:233). Active management of the third stage is recommended, particularly where there are concerns regarding coagulation and haemorrhage.

> ### Activity
> Why is ergometrine contraindicated in women with hypertension? How should the third stage of labour be managed?

Postnatal care
The mother

The risks of hypertensive disorders, including pre-eclampsia and eclampsia, continue after birth, particularly during the first 48 hours (Mol et al

2016). BP can rise after birth as uterine circulation decreases and fluid moves from the tissues into the general circulation (Heazell et al 2010). Postnatal BP peaks from around day 3 to day 6 (Magee et al 2014; McCarthy & Kenny 2015), when new hypertension may be observed. Any deterioration in end-organ function is most likely during this early postnatal period and in women with severe disease. Pre-eclampsia can appear for the first time within a few days of birth (Magee 2014), and eclampsia is most common postnatally (PROMPT Editorial Team 2017). Therefore continued close observation and monitoring of the woman's condition are essential, and continuing high-dependency care or hospitalization may be indicated. Anti-hypertensive medication will be reduced gradually to avoid rebound hypertension (McCarthy & Kenny 2015) and may be required for longer in women with pre-eclampsia than with gestational hypertension.

Activity

Why are non-steroidal anti-inflammatory drugs (NSAIDs) contra-indicated in women being treated for hypertension? What alternatives can be offered?

For most women with gestational hypertension and pre-eclampsia, the condition will have completely resolved by around 6 weeks following the birth (McCarthy & Kenny 2015). Therefore a medical review at 6 to 8 weeks post-birth should be offered to all women who have had these conditions (NICE 2010). Some women may require BP monitoring for 3 to 6 months (Cowan et al 2017). An individualized plan of care should be developed, documented and shared with the woman prior to her being discharged to and from community-based midwifery care.

The baby

Preterm birth is more likely for babies of women with gestational hypertensive disorders. Independent of prematurity, severe hypertension is associated with increased perinatal mortality and invasive ventilation, and pre-eclampsia increases the risk of bronchopulmonary dysplasia and necrotizing enterocolitis (Razak et al 2018). For premature babies who are small for gestational age, breast milk may offer some protection against hypertension in later life (Vargas-Martinez et al 2017), and NICE (2017:3) states that women can be reassured that anti-hypertensive drugs such as labetalol, nifedipine and atenolol have 'no known adverse effects on babies receiving breastmilk'. Midwives can support mothers and babies with feeding and skin contact as soon as possible to promote bonding and effective feeding. Where babies are born prematurely, mothers may require extra physical and emotional support in stimulating and maintaining milk production.

Gestational hypertension and pre-eclampsia may be associated with neurodevelopmental problems in childhood due to prematurity (Bokslag et al 2016). Children born to mothers with pre-eclampsia may also be more prone to poor growth and increased risk of hypertensive or cardiac disorders in later life (McCarthy & Kenny 2015).

Beyond the postnatal period

During the year following a pregnancy affected by hypertension, women are 12 to 25 times more likely to experience hypertension than women with normal pregnancy BP and 3 to 10 times more likely to have hypertension between 1 and 10 years (Behrens et al 2017). Women with pre-eclampsia are three to four times more likely to develop chronic hypertension; twice as likely to develop ischaemic heart disease, stroke or venous thromboembolism (Hutcheon et al 2011); and more likely to develop type 2 diabetes (Bokslag et al 2016). NICE (2010) recommends that women who have had pre-eclampsia should be advised that they have a 13% to 53% chance of gestational hypertension in future pregnancies and up to a 16% chance of pre-eclampsia recurring and that this increases to 25% if they had severe pre-eclampsia, HELLP syndrome or eclampsia. Where pre-eclampsia led to birth prior to 28 weeks' gestation, the chance of pre-eclampsia in a future pregnancy may be 55% (NICE 2010).

Prior to discharging women from their care, midwives can discuss the potential benefits of lifestyle changes and can, for example, signpost women to support in reducing their weight or smoking cessation (Mol et al 2016). Additionally, midwives can encourage women to attend follow-up care to identify and monitor ongoing hypertensive disorders with the aim of reducing the risk of complications (Behrens et al 2017).

Activity

Access the NICE Pathway for 'Hypertension in Pregnancy: Breastfeeding, Health Risks and Weight Management'. Think about how you might share this information with women in a supportive way.

Women's experiences of hypertensive disorders in pregnancy

A diagnosis of gestational hypertension or pre-eclampsia can surprise women, making them feel out of control and triggering fears for their personal or baby's wellbeing or guilt about their role in causing the condition. Women can lack clarity about the implications of their diagnosis until after the pregnancy has ended and they might be considering another pregnancy (Roberts et al 2017). Some women dislike taking high doses of medication, although 'tight' monitoring and control of hypertension can help women feel safe, and being well informed helps women to accept treatment and feel satisfied with their care (Vidler et al 2016). Trusting care providers is important in feeling safe and can be enhanced by clear communication and continuity of care and carer (Roberts et al 2017), highlighting the importance of effective multi-disciplinary and individualized care.

REFLECTION ON THE TRIGGER SCENARIO

Look back on the trigger scenario.

Olivia is 42 years old and following her second cycle of IVF. She discovers that she is pregnant for the first time. Whilst she is overjoyed, she is also concerned that as an older pregnant woman, she and her baby have a greater chance of complications such as hypertension. Her blood pressure is borderline, and with a family history of hypertension, she has read a lot about these potential risk factors. Olivia wants to be as involved as possible in decision-making about the care and management of her pregnancy.

The scenario is one that highlights the importance of involving women in their care and factors that might pre-dispose women to a pregnancy that is complicated by hypertensive disorders. Now that you are familiar with the issues in relation to hypertension in pregnancy, you should have insight into how the scenario relates to the evidence. The jigsaw model will now be used to explore the trigger scenario in more depth.

Effective communication

Effective identification, investigation, management and support for women with hypertensive disorders in pregnancy can involve complex issues. Therefore, it can be challenging for midwives to be sure that women have a sufficient understanding about their condition to make valid choices about their care. Questions that arise from this scenario might include: What questions could the midwife ask Olivia to establish her prior understanding about hypertensive disorders?

How could Olivia's responses enhance information-sharing? What methods can the midwife use to ensure that Olivia understands any new information?

Woman-centred care

Hypertensive disorders in pregnancy vary significantly. Similarly, women's responses to being informed about threats to their personal health or their baby's health will be determined by a range of factors such as their cultural and medical backgrounds. Questions that may be asked in relation to this scenario are: How might continuity of care from a known midwife benefit Olivia in addition to reviews with a consultant obstetrician? What support networks does Olivia have, and how can these help Olivia feel safe? How can the midwife ensure that she is meeting Olivia's physical, emotional and social needs?

Using best evidence

Due to the limited time frame of pregnancy and ethical considerations in relation to drug trials in pregnancy, pre-eclampsia is difficult to research, but the body of evidence about hypertensive disorders in pregnancy is developing (Cowan et al 2017). Questions that arise from the scenario might include: How can midwives ensure that the information they share with women is the most relevant to women's needs? If a woman presents with symptoms of pre-eclampsia but does not have hypertension or proteinuria, what actions should be taken? In what circumstances might women request care that is outside the current guidelines? Does Olivia have access to written information about hypertensive disorders in pregnancy?

Professional and legal issues

Midwives are responsible for practising in accordance with the Code (Nursing and Midwifery Council (NMC) 2015), their employer's policies and the law. Providing high-quality care for women with potentially life-threatening conditions such as pre-eclampsia requires adequate resources. Questions that arise from the scenario might include: In what ways can detailed, contemporaneous documentation support professional and accountable midwifery care? How does the use of Maternity Early Warning Scoring (MEWS) systems enable midwives to ensure that they respond appropriately to the woman's clinical assessment? What would be the midwife's responsibilities if Olivia declined investigations or treatments in relation to hypertensive disorders?

Team working

Providing safe and effective care in relation to complex needs such as hypertension involves close liaison between the members of the multi-professional team, regardless of whether they have direct or indirect contact with the woman. Questions that could arise from the scenario include: Which clinical disciplines might be involved in the care of a woman with hypertension? How can midwives ensure that relevant investigations are carried out and the results acted upon in a timely manner? What are the potential benefits of using a structured approach, such as Situation, Background, Assessment, Recommendation (SBAR), to sharing information about women's needs? In what circumstances might the midwife need to escalate Olivia's care to another health professional?

Clinical dexterity

Midwives are responsible for ensuring that maternal observations such as BP measurements and urinalysis are performed accurately and appropriately and that any concerns are escalated in a timely manner. Similarly, assessing fetal wellbeing is a key midwifery role. Questions that might arise in relation to Olivia's situation include: What factors should be considered before measuring a woman's BP to ensure that the reading is accurate? What are the key clinical considerations that need to be combined in the assessment of Olivia's obstetric health and emotional wellbeing? How could the use of an individualized fetal growth chart help the midwife detect fetal growth restriction or oligohydramnios?

Models of care

Women who have hypertensive disorders in pregnancy are likely to experience multi-professional care. However, they still need to experience care that is woman-centred and personal. Questions that arise from the scenario might include: Why is midwifery-led care inappropriate for women with complex needs? How might continuity of carer benefit women, such as Olivia, who might have appointments with a number of different health professionals? How could midwifery care be organized so that Olivia is cared for by a familiar midwife in the hospital setting? How can 'white coat' hypertension be avoided?

Safe environment

Midwives have a responsibility to 'protect patient and public safety' (NMC 2015). They need to ensure that women feel emotionally secure as well as in safe clinical hands. Questions that arise from the scenario might include: If midwives are concerned about the care of women with hypertension that has been ordered by junior doctors, what actions should they take? What are the advantages and disadvantages of women with pre-eclampsia giving birth to their baby in an obstetric unit? What equipment should the midwife ensure is checked and available to her when caring for a woman with pre-eclampsia?

Promotes health

Promoting health is a key midwifery responsibility and, in relation to the detection and management of hypertensive disorders in pregnancy, involves assessing and managing risk, sharing information and providing physical care for the mother and baby. Questions that arise from the scenario might include: How might women's lifestyle affect their potential for hypertension-related maternal and perinatal morbidity and mortality? With regard to the future, what information and support could be provided postnatally to women whose pregnancy has been affected by hypertension?

Further scenarios

The following scenarios enable you to consider how specific situations influence the care the midwife provides. Use the jigsaw model to explore the issues raised in the scenario.

SCENARIO 1

Alya is 33 weeks pregnant in her second pregnancy and has been admitted to the antenatal ward with pre-eclampsia. Alya was diagnosed with pre-eclampsia during her first pregnancy, and after being born at 32 weeks' gestation, her baby was cared for on the neonatal unit for 4 weeks and then on the transitional care unit. Alya is worried that this will happen again and wonders how she will cope with caring for a sick baby in hospital and her young daughter at home.

Practice point

Alya's situation highlights the risk of pre-eclampsia occurring in subsequent pregnancies and the potential for hypertensive disorders to pose emotional and social challenges. The stresses and concerns experienced by pregnant women with hypertension may go far beyond their current pregnancy. Previous experiences can influence expectations and provoke anxieties impacting on choices and decision-making.

Questions that could be asked are:

1. How might Alya's risk of pre-eclampsia have been reduced for her current pregnancy?
2. What prophylaxis could be offered to reduce the risk of Alya's baby having respiratory difficulties after birth?
3. If Alya's baby requires care on a neonatal unit, how can she be supported in feeding and building a relationship with her baby?
4. How can Alya's daughter be prepared for the early arrival of her sibling?
5. Where might Alya's care be transferred to if there were no neonatal cots available in her local maternity unit?

SCENARIO 2

Two days after a routine 28-week appointment with her community midwife, Chloe wakens from sleep with a throbbing headache and feeling nauseated. She takes paracetamol and goes back to bed. After a couple of hours her headache feels worse and she starts vomiting. She catches sight of herself in the mirror and notices that her face is very swollen. She remembers discussing the signs of pre-eclampsia with her midwife.

Practice point

Chloe's situation demonstrates the potential for the sudden onset of hypertensive disorders and the importance of sharing information with women about the signs and symptoms of pre-eclampsia. Chloe requires urgent care and immediate admission to a maternity unit and senior obstetric review.

Questions that could be asked are:

1. How can midwives share information about pre-eclampsia without causing undue anxiety for pregnant women?
2. How clear is the information provided to women about how and when to contact a midwife or doctor for help and advice?
3. What advice should be given to Chloe in this situation?
4. Where should she attend for care?
5. How should she travel?
6. What preparations might the multi-disciplinary team make for Chloe's imminent admission?

Conclusion

Hypertensive disorders in pregnancy are associated with a range of risk factors; they vary in presentation and severity and have the potential to cause adverse short- and long-term outcomes for mother and baby. Women can present with hypertensive disorders at any stage during their pregnancy, before, during or after the birth of their baby. Therefore, midwives are in a prime position to identify the risk factors, signs and symptoms of hypertensive disorders; to refer women for specialist care; and to provide information that will help them understand what these disorders and any proposed management might mean for them. Through developing and maintaining effective relationships with women and their families and other members of the multi-disciplinary team, midwives can help build trust, enhancing women's experiences and the effectiveness of care, with the potential to improve outcomes for mothers and their babies.

Resources

Action on Pre-Eclampsia (APEC)

Information and e-learning resource available at: https://action-on-pre-eclampsia. org.uk/

British Heart Foundation

Funds research into cardiovascular diseases, and provides resources for health professionals. Available at: https://www.bhf.org.uk/for-professionals

NICE (2010) Hypertension in pregnancy: diagnosis and management: Clinical Guideline 107. Available at: https://www.nice.org.uk/guidance/cg107

Royal College of Obstetricians and Gynaecologists

Information for women and their families about pre-eclampsia. Available at: https:// www.rcog.org.uk/globalassets/documents/patients/patient-information-leaflets/pregnancy/pi-pre-eclampsia.pdf

Tommy's

Information for parents and health professionals available at: https://www. tommys.org/pregnancy-information/pregnancy-complications/pre-eclampsia-information-and-support

World Health Organization (WHO)

WHO (2011) Recommendations for Prevention and Treatment of Pre-Eclampsia and Eclampsia. Available at: https://www.ncbi.nlm.nih.gov/books/NBK140560/#ch4.s8

References

Baston, H., Hall, J., 2017. Midwifery Essentials: Basics, second ed. Elsevier, London.

Baston, H., Hall, J., 2018. Midwifery Essentials: Emergency Maternity Care, vol. 6. Elsevier, London.

Behrens, I., Basit, S., Melbye, M., et al., 2017. Risk of post-pregnancy hypertension in women with a history of hypertensive disorders of pregnancy: nationwide cohort study. BMJ 358 (j3078), https://doi.org/10.1136/bmj.j3078.

Bokslag, A., van Weissenbruch, M., Mol, B.W., de Groot, C.J.M., 2016. Pre-eclampsia; short and long-term consequences for mother and neonate. Early Hum. Dev. 102, 47–50. http://dx.doi.org/10.1016/j.earlhumdev.2016.09.007.

Bramham, K., Parnell, B., Nelson-Piercy, C., et al., 2014. Chronic hypertension and pregnancy outcomes: systematic review and meta-analysis. BMJ 348 (g2301), https://doi.org/10.1136/bmj.g2301.

British Heart Foundation, 2018. CVD Fact Sheet. Available from: https://www.bhf.org.uk/for-professionals/press-centre/facts-and-figures.

Bujold, E., Roberge, S., Lacasse, Y., et al., 2010. Prevention of preeclampsia and intrauterine growth restriction with aspirin started in early pregnancy: a meta-analysis. Obstet. Gynecol. 116 (2 Parr 1), doi:10.1097/AOG.0b013e3181e9322a.

CLASP (Collaborative Low-dose Aspirin Study in Pregnancy) Collaborative Group, 1994. CLASP: a randomised trial of low-dose aspirin for the prevention and treatment of pre-eclampsia among 9364 pregnant women. Lancet 343, 619–629. https://doi.org/10.1016/S0140-6736(94)92633-6.

Connolly, K.A., Factor, S.H., Getrajdman, C.S., et al., 2016. Maternal clinical disease characteristics and maternal and neonatal outcomes in twin and singleton pregnancies with severe pre-eclampsia. Eur. J. Obstet. Gynecol. Reprod. Biol. 201, 36–41. http://dx.doi.org/10.1016/j.ejogrb.2015.11.031.

Cowan, J., Redman, C., Walker, I., 2017. Understanding Pre-Eclampsia. Clearsay Publishing, Watford.

Daskas, N., Crowne, E., Shield, J.P.H., 2013. Is labetalol really a culprit in neonatal hypoglycaemia? Arch. Dis. Child. Fetal Neonatal Ed. http://dx.doi.org/10.1136/archdischild-2012-303057.

De Ocampo, M.P.G., Araneta, M.R.G., Macera, C.A., et al., 2018. Folic acid supplement use and the risk of gestational hypertension and preeclampsia. Women Birth 31, e77–e83. http://dx.doi.org/10.1016/j.wombi.2017.08.128.

Eclampsia Trial Collaborative Group, 1995. Which anti-convulsant for women with eclampsia? Evidence from the Collaborative Eclampsia Trial. Lancet 345, 1455–1463. https://doi.org/10.5555/uri:pii:S0140673695910344.

Ferrazzani, S., Moresi, S., De Feo, E., et al., 2015. Is gestational hypertension beneficial in twin pregnancies? Pregnancy Hypertens. 5, 171–176. http://dx.doi.org/10.1016/j.preghy.2015.01.003.

Harding, K., Redmond, P., Tuffnell, D., on behalf of the MBRRACE-UK Hypertensive disorders of pregnancy chapter writing group, 2016. Caring for women with hypertensive disorders of pregnancy. In: Knight, M., Nour, M., Tuffnell, D., et al. on behalf of MBRRACE-UK (Eds.), Saving Lives, Improving Mothers' Care – Surveillance of Maternal Deaths in the UK 2012-14 and Lessons Learned to Inform Maternity Care From the UK and Ireland Confidential Enquiries Into Maternal Deaths and Morbidity 2009-14. National Perinatal Epidemiology Unit, University of Oxford, Oxford, pp. 69–75. Available from: https://www.npeu.ox.ac.uk/downloads/files/mbrrace-uk/reports/MBRRACE-UK%20Maternal%20Report%202016%20-%20website.pdf.

Heazell, A., Evans, K., 2017. Antenatal care. In: Draper, E.S., Kurinczuk, J.J., Kenyon, S., on behalf of MBRRACE-UK (Eds.), MBRRACE-UK 2017 Perinatal Confidential Enquiry: Term, Singleton, Intrapartum Stillbirth and Intrapartum-Related Neonatal Death. The Infant Mortality and Morbidity

Studies, Department of Health Sciences, University of Leicester, Leicester, pp. 67–72. Available from: https://www.npeu.ox.ac.uk/downloads/files/mbrrace-uk/reports/MBRRACE-UK%20Intrapartum%20Confidential%20Enquiry%20Report%202017%20-%20final%20version.pdf.

Heazell, A., Norwitz, E.R., Kenny, L.C., Baker, P.N. (Eds.), 2010. Hypertension in Pregnancy. Cambridge University Press, Cambridge.

Hutcheon, J.A., Lisonkova, S., Joseph, K.S., 2011. Epidemiology of pre-eclampsia and the other hypertensive disorders of pregnancy. Best Pract. Res. Clin. Obstet. Gynaecol. 25, 391–403. doi:10.1016/j.bpobgyn.2011.01.006.

Kourtis, A., 2012. Diabetes and gestational hypertension. Curr. Hypertens. Rev. 8, 127–129.

Magee, L.A., Pels, A., Helewa, M., et al. on behalf of the Canadian Hypertensive Disorders of Pregnancy (HDP) Group, 2014. Diagnosis, evaluation and management of the hypertensive disorders of pregnancy. Pregnancy Hypertens. 4, 105–145. http://dx.doi.org/10.1016/j.preghy.2014.01.003.

McCarthy, F., Kenny, L.C., 2015. Hypertension in pregnancy. Obstet. Gynaecol. Reprod. Med. 25 (8), 229–235. doi:10.1016/j.ogrm.2015.05.004.

McCarthy, F.P., Kenny, L.C., 2010. Adaptations of maternal cardiovascular and renal physiology to pregnancy. In: Heazell, A., Norwitz, E.R., Kenny, L.C., Baker, P.N. (Eds.), Hypertension in Pregnancy. Cambridge University Press, Cambridge, pp. 1–18.

McLeod, L., 2008. How useful is uterine artery Doppler ultrasonography in predicting pre-eclampsia and intrauterine growth restriction? Can. Med J. Assoc. 178 (6), https://doi.org/10.1503/cmaj.080242.

Mol, B.W.J., Thangaratinam, S., Magee, L.A., et al., 2016. Pre-eclampsia. Lancet 387, 999–1011. doi:10.1016/S0140-6736(15)00070-7.

National Institute for Health and Care Excellence, 2010. Hypertension in Pregnancy: Diagnosis and Management. Available from: https://www.nice.org.uk/guidance/cg107.

National Institute for Health and Care Excellence, 2017. Hypertension in pregnancy: breastfeeding, health risks and weight management. Available from: http://pathways.nice.org.uk/pathways/hypertension-in-pregnancy.

Nursing and Midwifery Council, 2015. The Code: Professional standards of practice and behaviour for nurses and midwives. Available from: https://www.nmc.org.uk/globalassets/sitedocuments/nmc-publications/nmc-code.pdf.

Pieper, P.G., Hoendermis, E.S., 2011. Pregnancy in women with pulmonary hypertension. Neth. Heart J. 19, 504–508. doi:10.1007/s12471-011-0219-9.

PROMPT Editorial Team, 2017. PROMPT Course Manual, third ed. Cambridge University Press, Cambridge.

Razak, A., Florendo-Chin, A., Banfield, L., et al., 2018. Pregnancy-induced hypertension and neonatal outcomes: a systematic review and meta-analysis. J. Perinatol. 38, 46–53. doi:10.1038/jp.2017.162.

Repke, J.T., Norwitz, E.R., 2010. Management in eclampsia. In: Heazell, A., Norwitz, E.R., Kenny, L.C., Baker, P.N. (Eds.), (2010) Hypertension in Pregnancy. Cambridge University Press, Cambridge, pp. 141–158.

Roberts, L.M., Davis, G.K., Homer, C.S.E., 2017. Pregnancy with gestational hypertension or preeclampsia: a qualitative exploration of women's experiences. Midwifery 46, 17–23. http://dx.doi.org/10.1016/j.midw.2017.01.004.

Royal College of Obstetricians and Gynaecologists (RCOG), 2015. Reducing the risk of venous thromboembolism during pregnancy and the puerperium: Greentop Guideline 37a. Available from: https://www.rcog.org.uk/globalassets/documents/guidelines/gtg-37a.pdf.

Ryan, R.M., McCarthy, F.P., 2018. Hypertension in Pregnancy. Obstet. Gynaecol. Reprod. Med. 28 (5), 141–147. doi:10.1016/j.ogrm.2018.03.003.

Traquilli, A.L., Dekker, G., Magee, I., et al., 2014. The classification, diagnosis and management of the hypertensive disorders of pregnancy: a revised statement from the International Society for the Study of Hypertension in Pregnancy (ISSHP). Pregnancy Hypertens. 4, 97–104. https://doi.org/10.1016/j.preghy.2014.02.001.

Ukah, U.V., De Silva, D.A., Payne, B., et al., 2018. Prediction of adverse maternal outcomes from pre-eclampsia and other hypertensive disorders of pregnancy: a systematic review. Pregnancy Hypertens. 11, 115–123. https://doi.org/10.1016/j.preghy.2017.11.006.

Vargas-Martínez, F., Schanler, R.J., Abrams, S.A., et al., 2017. Oxytocin, a main breastfeeding hormone, prevents hypertension acquired in utero: a therapeutics preview. Biochim. Biophys. Acta 1861 (1), 3071–3084. doi:10.1016/j.bbagen.2016.09.020.

Vidler, M., Magee, L.A., von Dadelszen, P., et al. the The CHIPS Study Group, 2016. Women's views and postpartum follow-up in the CHIPS Trial (Control of Hypertension in Pregnancy Study). Eur. J. Obstet. Gynaecol. Reprod. Biol. 206, 105–113. doi:10.1016/j.ejogrb.2016.07.509.

CHAPTER 4

Respiratory disorders in childbearing

TRIGGER SCENARIO

Chantelle is 17 years old and has had asthma since she was 6 years old. Many of her close family are cigarette smokers, and she began smoking at age 14. She has had regular inhaler medication prescribed for her asthma, although she doesn't always remember to use the preventer. She is unsure about whether using her inhaler could harm her baby so has only used it on a couple of occasions, even though she has felt breathless at times. Chantelle is anxious about arranging a booking appointment, thinking that she will probably be criticized for smoking.

Introduction

In the United Kingdom respiratory diseases account for around 19% of all deaths in women; these respiratory-related deaths are linked with a number of factors such as smoking and socio-economic deprivation. Furthermore, approximately 10,000 people are given new diagnoses of respiratory diseases each week (British Lung Foundation 2018). Therefore, midwives are highly likely to come into contact with women who have pre-existing respiratory disease, such as asthma or cystic fibrosis (CF), or who develop new conditions, such as pneumonia, during pregnancy or the postnatal period. Whilst midwives may not have the expertise to take a lead in caring for these women, having an understanding of how respiratory disorders can impact on the experiences and outcomes of childbearing women, their babies and their families will help them to coordinate and contribute to safe care and management. This chapter briefly summarizes the physiological adaptations to respiration during pregnancy and outlines the presentation, treatment and pregnancy-related issues for women with asthma, CF, pneumonia, tuberculosis (TB) and sarcoidosis. Emergency respiratory collapse is covered in Chapter 1, Volume 6 (Baston & Hall 2018) and influenza is addressed in Chapter 8 of this volume.

Respiratory system adaptations in pregnancy and childbearing

Changes in the anatomy and physiology of respiration are essential during pregnancy to accommodate the increased metabolic demands associated with physical changes within the woman's body and the additional demands of the developing placenta and fetus (Rankin 2017). Hormonal, metabolic and mechanical factors drive these changes (Bhatia et al 2016). In the upper respiratory tract, blood flow to the nasal mucosa increases, increasing the occurrence of epistaxis. The chest cavity changes in shape, becoming wider and flatter as the diaphragm is pushed upwards and the intercostals muscles relax; breathing becomes more thoracic than abdominal (Rankin 2017). Fig. 4.1 demonstrates the pregnancy-related changes in the mother's chest shape.

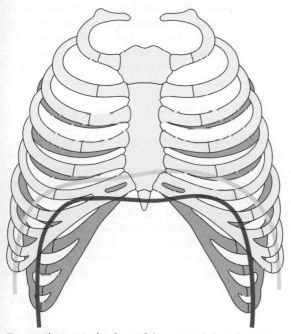

Fig. 4.1 Changes in the shape of the maternal chest during pregnancy. (From Rankin J: Respiration In: Rankin J (Ed) Physiology in Childbearing with Anatomy and Related Biosciences (pp 183-194). London: Elsevier–figure 18.9)

During pregnancy, the demand for oxygen increases by around 16% supplied by an increase in ventilation of the lungs of approximately 40%. The respiratory rate remains largely the same as pre-pregnancy; however, the volume of breaths (tidal volume) increases by around 200 ml (Rankin 2017). Carbon dioxide saturation levels are lower, causing a slight respiratory alkalosis. This is partly due to the increase in ventilation (Bhatia et al 2016). Pregnant women can experience dyspnoea or shortness of breath, which can be worse if they are sitting (Rankin 2017). Fetal oxygenation is dependent on maternal oxygenation of the placenta and placental transfer (Bhatia et al 2016).

Respiratory disorders and maternal mortality

During 2013–2015 in the United Kingdom, there were 43 maternal deaths resulting from medical or general surgical issues, and 9 of these deaths were related to respiratory disorders. This included two deaths from asthma and two from CF, and for some women who died from known lung disease, pulmonary hypertension was an element of their condition (Knight & Nelson-Piercy 2017). Not all of these women received pre- and post-pregnancy counselling about their condition or contraceptive advice, even when they had already experienced a high-risk pregnancy. When women had been provided with advice about their respiratory condition in relation to pregnancy, it was not always clear that women understood what had been said to them (Knight & Nelson-Piercy 2017).

Asthma

Asthma is a relatively common chronic respiratory condition that features reversible and intermittent narrowing of the airways, inflammation and reactivity to a number of stimulants, such as respiratory tract infections, pollen, dust mites, cold air, tobacco and some drugs (such as aspirin, non-steroidal anti-inflammatory drugs and β-blockers) (National Institute for Health and Care Excellence (NICE) 2017a; Stephen & Teirstein 2013). It may be linked with atopic conditions such as eczema and allergic rhinitis (Stephen & Teirstein 2013). The impact of asthma varies but is characterized by exacerbations or attacks of wheezing and breathlessness, which if severe can be life threatening (NICE 2017a).

Assessment and diagnosis of asthma

Diagnosing asthma can be difficult, as there is 'no gold standard test' (NICE 2017a). Where asthma is suspected, a structured clinical assessment is required to exclude alternative diagnoses.

+ History taking using a validated questionnaire is likely to include reports of:
  + Wheezing, cough or dyspnoea (symptoms may be worse at night)
  + Personal or family history of atopic conditions (British Thoracic Society and Scottish Intercollegiate Guidelines Network (BTSSIGN) 2016; Stephen & Teirstein 2013).
+ Chest auscultation by a health professional confirms the presence of a wheeze.
+ Airway inflammation testing measuring fractional exhaled nitric oxide (FENO) is increasingly used in diagnosing asthma and may help guide corticosteroid use (Morten et al 2018).
+ Lung function and airflow are assessed using spirometry and peak expiratory flow (PEF) monitors; spirometry can be combined with bronchodilator-reversibility assessments (BTSSIGN 2016; NICE 2017a).

Management of asthma

Asthma management involves both non-pharmacological and pharmacological interventions. The aims of treatment are to:

+ Control the symptoms and promote normal lung functioning
+ Improve the quality of life
+ Minimize the side effects of medications

Non-pharmacological strategies

These include encouraging self-management, which can improve asthma control and reduce the need for emergency care (BTSSIGN 2016). Education about asthma and developing and regularly evaluating a personal asthma action plan (PAAP) with asthma specialists are central to self-care. PAAPs should include a cohesive drug regimen, actions women should take if their asthma deteriorates or in an emergency, avoidance of triggers, support with smoking cessation or weight loss (if appropriate) and breathing exercises (Asthma UK 2016; BTSSIGN 2016). Self-management might also promote a greater sense of control.

Pharmacological management

Drug therapy in asthma management involves the use of a stepwise approach to prescribing drugs according to individual needs; medications are stepped up when greater control is required and vice versa. Treatment commonly includes reliever and preventive medications.

+ Intermittent reliever therapy: Inhaled bronchodilators (short-acting β_2 agonists (SABAs)) such as salbutamol relieve the symptoms of asthma and are not associated with adverse perinatal outcomes.

+ Regular preventer therapy: Inhaled corticosteroids (ICSs) such as beclomethasone improve asthma symptoms and lung functioning; they decrease the risk of asthma attacks in pregnancy and are not associated with adverse perinatal outcomes. Smoking reduces the effectiveness of ICSs (BTSSIGN 2016).

Additional drugs, such as oral steroids or long-acting β_2 agonists (LABAs), may be required when asthma is severe, and involving asthma specialists may be indicated (BTSSIGN 2016).

Asthma and pregnancy

Most pregnant women with asthma do not experience associated complications, particularly where the condition is well controlled, and in some cases, asthma improves during pregnancy. However, asthma and pregnancy *can* affect each other, and up to one-fifth of pregnant women with asthma are likely to need urgent management for acute symptoms at some point; the risk is higher with severe disease. Severe symptoms are most common around the sixth month of pregnancy. Poorly controlled asthma is associated with hypertensive diseases in pregnancy, haemorrhage, preterm labour and birth, low birth weight, perinatal hypoxia and mortality (BTSSIGN 2016). Asthma attacks are uncommon during late pregnancy, labour and birth because of high cortisol levels around these times (Mehta et al 2015).

Pregnancy care

In addition to routine pregnancy care, midwives can encourage women with asthma to continue to regularly review their PAAP, including their medication regimen, with their asthma nurse or specialist. Midwives are also responsible for ensuring that the plan is incorporated into maternity records and shared with the maternity multi-disciplinary team. Fear about the effects of medication on their baby may lead to non-compliance; by encouraging pregnant women to continue with asthma medication as normal, midwives can promote good asthma control and help avoid complications (BTSSIGN 2016; Mehta et al 2015), including maternal death (Knight & Nelson-Piercy 2017). Commonly used asthma medication is generally considered safe in pregnancy, since the risks of poorly controlled asthma outweigh small risks from the medication (BTSSIGN 2016).

Two of the women whose asthma-related deaths were reported by Knight and Nelson-Piercy (2017) were smokers. Midwives are in an ideal position to refer women who smoke for smoking cessation support (Marshall & Baston 2019) and to involve the woman's family in discussing what to do in case of an asthma attack (Asthma UK 2016).

Fetal wellbeing can be assessed using ultrasonography to measure growth (Stephen & Teirstein 2013), and electronic fetal monitoring is indicated for women with severe asthma during pregnancy and labour in accordance with the mother's condition (BTSSIGN 2016).

Emergency care

Acute severe asthma in pregnancy is an emergency, and management is the same as for someone who is not pregnant. This includes administering oxygen to achieve saturation at 94% to 98% and may involve oral or intravenous medications. Urgent involvement of critical care or respiratory teams may be necessary (BTSSIGN 2016).

Labour care

Whilst asthma attacks in labour are rare, there are labour-specific considerations in caring for women with asthma:

- During labour, women with asthma can safely use the usual pain-relieving methods, and using E_2 prostaglandins is safe for the induction of labour.
- Carboprost (Hemabate), used in the management of postpartum haemorrhage and ergometrine, can cause bronchospasm and should only be used with extreme caution.
- Regional anaesthetic is preferable to general anaesthetic when this is required.
- Caesarean birth is associated with increased postnatal asthma attacks (BTSSIGN 2016).

Postnatal care

Following birth, women with asthma should be supported to breastfeed and can continue to take asthma medications in accordance with drug manufacturers' recommendations (BTSSIGN 2016). Breastfeeding may reduce the chance of the baby developing asthma when older (Asthma UK 2016), particularly if breastfeeding extends beyond 4 months.

Activity

Find out more about FENO tests, spirometry and PEF measurements. What is the difference between an inhaler device and a nebulizer? When might each be indicated?

Cystic fibrosis

In the United Kingdom Caucasian population, CF is the most common life-threatening genetic disorder. This genetic defect in the CF transmembrane conductance regulator (CFTR) is autosomal recessive (Stephen & Teirstein 2013). It is associated with epithelial and mucous gland dysfunction, resulting in thickened secretions, obstruction and organ failure (Kroon et al 2018). CF is a multi-system disorder with many mutations; it affects mainly the lungs, sinuses, sweat glands and digestive system but can also involve the liver, joints and male fertility. Less commonly, it is linked with meconium ileus (Stephen & Teirstein 2013) and diabetes (National Consensus Standards for the Nursing Management of Cystic Fibrosis (NCSNMCF) 2016). Morbidity and mortality result most frequently from chronic and degenerative respiratory disease, complicated by recurrent infections (Stephen & Teirstein 2013). Weight gain and maintenance can be problematic due to pancreatic insufficiency, malabsorption and increased energy expenditure (Ahluwalia et al 2014). The establishment of CF specialist teams, improvements in anti-microbial treatment, nutritional care, mucous clearance and newborn screening have increased the life expectancy of people with CF over recent years (Kroon et al 2018). Consequently, more females with CF are likely to reach childbearing age, and since CF has little impact on female fertility, midwives are increasingly likely to be involved in their care (Ahluwalia et al 2014; Kroon et al 2018).

Cystic fibrosis and pregnancy

With good pre-conception care, pregnant women with CF are unlikely to experience adverse immediate or medium-term outcomes and, unless specific problems are identified, can expect to birth their baby vaginally (Stephen & Teirstein 2013). Ongoing support from a multi-disciplinary team is important, including obstetricians, midwives, respiratory physicians, specialist nurses, physiotherapists, nutritionists, pharmacists and clinical psychologists (NICE 2017b).

Severe CF with right-sided heart and pancreatic involvement is associated with increases in premature birth, antibiotic requirements, hospitalization, morbidity and mortality. Lung function and chest physiotherapy can be compromised as pregnancy advances, some women have difficulty gaining weight and there is an increased risk of gestational diabetes (Ahluwalia et al 2014). The risk of teratogenicity limits the options for antibiotic therapy. For example, tetracyclines can cause bone and tooth discolouration; trimethoprim is associated with neural tube defects and neonatal icterus (Stephen & Teirstein 2013). However, Kroon et al (2018) suggest that primary consideration must be for the mother's health rather than the fetus or neonate.

Midwives may have little direct involvement in managing women's CF care but can help women understand the need for obstetric and ongoing

CF specialist team management, can listen to their concerns and can provide support regarding other aspects of their pregnancy, birth and becoming a mother. Providing postnatal information about contraception is an important aspect of ongoing care (NICE 2017b).

Activity

What information can you give to a woman with CF regarding the risk of her baby being affected by the condition?

Find out which health professionals are likely to be involved in caring for people with CF.

Pneumonia

Pneumonia is an infection of the lower respiratory tract (below the larynx) and can develop as a result of inhalation, aspiration, blood-borne or traumatic transmission (Preston & Kelly 2016). The infection can be bacterial, viral or fungal in origin (Stephen & Teirstein 2013). Pneumonia causes inflammation of lung alveoli, which impairs gaseous exchange (Preston & Kelly 2016). Symptoms include fever, cough, dyspnoea and varying degrees of hypoxia (Mehta et al 2015). Whilst some degree of dyspnoea is relatively normal during pregnancy, tachypnoea is not, and any evidence of this requires further investigation (Stephen & Teirstein 2013). Lung consolidation (the presence of dense material such as fluid or pus rather than air) on chest X-ray is indicative of pneumonia (Preston & Kelly 2016). People who are smokers or have co-existing disorders such as HIV, CF and asthma have an increased chance of developing pneumonia.

Pneumonia in pregnancy

Respiratory changes in pregnancy mean that pregnant women are also vulnerable to pneumonia and potential complications, such as septic shock (Mehta et al 2015). Whilst pneumonia is not common in pregnancy (Stephen & Teirstein 2013), there is an increased risk of severe disease, need for ventilatory support in an intensive care setting and higher incidence of pre-eclampsia (Kriebs 2015). It is associated with higher rates of intervention during labour, and caesarean birth increases the potential for postnatal pneumonia (Mehta et al 2015). Possible effects on the fetus include preterm rupture of membranes and prematurity, intrauterine growth restriction and hypoxaemia secondary to maternal hypoxia (Kriebs 2015). Bacterial pneumonia is treated with antibiotics such as cephalosporins, which are safe in pregnancy, and anti-viral medications are used to treat viral pneumonia (Mehta et al 2015).

Tuberculosis

TB is a droplet-borne infection most commonly caused by *Mycobacterium tuberculosis*. Historically referred to as *consumption*, TB is associated with overcrowded or poor living conditions and poor general health (Dyer 2010; Public Health England (PHE) 2018). In the 1980s rates rose by around 65%, most notably amongst people with suppressed immunity, for instance, as a result of HIV or AIDS (Barnett 2018). TB can cause life-threatening disease and almost exclusively affects the lungs in the UK (PHE 2018) but can spread to other organs (Dyer 2010), such as the genitourinary tract and bone (Stephen & Teirstein 2013).

Infection with TB does not always follow exposure, and of people who become infected, around 10% will develop active TB within a couple of years (Dyer 2010). As the body attempts to fight off the infection firm grey lesions (tubercles) form, damaging lung or other affected tissue and forming scars which trap the bacteria; this is called *latent infection*. If the immune response cannot contain the infection, active TB ensues. Early signs include coughing, which is sometimes blood-stained (haemoptysis) if capillaries are damaged (Dyer 2010). As more lung tissue is affected, breathing becomes increasingly difficult; the person becomes fatigued and experiences weight loss (PHE 2013). Whilst TB is treatable, worldwide it is one of the leading causes of infection-related deaths (Dyer 2010).

TB in pregnancy

Pregnancy affects women's immunity to infection, increasing their vulnerability to active TB disease. TB in pregnancy can progress quickly, particularly if women also have HIV or are otherwise compromised (Bates et al 2015; PHE 2013). Where TB is diagnosed and treatment commenced early in pregnancy, the prognosis is good. However, symptoms of pulmonary TB can mimic symptoms of pregnancy (breathlessness and fatigue), leading to treatment delays and increasing the potential for morbidity and premature labour (PHE 2013).

Investigations

History taking can reveal that a pregnant woman is at high risk of TB infection, for example, through having HIV or close contact with someone who has TB, and clinical assessment may indicate possible infection. Either scenario requires investigation for evidence of infection (PHE 2013). Table 4.1 outlines investigations used to diagnose TB infection.

Table 4.1: **Investigations to diagnose tuberculosis**

- **Tuberculin skin test (TST):** The standard test is the Mantoux test, whereby purified protein derivative (PPD) of *Mycobacterium tuberculosis* is injected into the skin; a positive test – local redness and swelling – indicates infection with TB but does not differentiate between latent and active infection. PPD is non-infectious (PHE 2013).
- **Interferon gamma release assay (IGRA) blood test:** May be performed concurrently with the TST (NICE 2016), and if these tests are positive, the woman should be investigated for active TB.
- **Chest X-ray:** Diagnostic testing for pulmonary TB includes a chest X-ray to determine whether infection is active (protection of the maternal abdomen is required to protect the developing fetus).
- **Sputum samples:** Multiple samples should be tested for TB microscopy and culture; rapid diagnostic nucleic acid amplification tests can be requested if the woman has HIV or specific information is required to inform treatment (NICE 2016). The tubercle bacilli take 8 weeks to grow (Stephen & Teirstein 2013).

Treatment

Specialist multi-disciplinary working is essential in managing TB in pregnancy by educating women about TB, conducting the investigations and developing an individualized plan, which includes treatment and offering screening to close contacts (NICE 2016). Effective treatment normally comprises multiple antibiotics, which help to prevent drug resistance; treatment needs to be continued for around 6 to 9 months (Dyer 2010).

- Prophylactic treatment with isoniazid (INH), or INH with rifampicin, can be given to pregnant women who are considered high risk and whose skin or blood tests were positive but do not have symptoms or evidence of TB on chest X-ray (PHE 2013).
- Where women are diagnosed with active TB, the aim of treatment is to cure the infection and prevent its spread (PHE 2013). Women with active disease are offered treatment with first-line anti-TB drugs: INH, rifampicin, pyrazinamide and ethambutol (PHE 2013). Often INH and rifampicin are the only drugs continued beyond 2 months. Although INH crosses the placenta during pregnancy (Stephen & Teirstein 2013), treatment during pregnancy is not linked with major toxicity in the mother or fetus (Bates et al 2015).

Pulmonary TB is not normally infectious after 2 weeks of treatment with INH and rifampicin (PHE 2013). Midwives and other health workers have a responsibility to work within local guidelines for limiting the spread of infection, and this may involve caring for the woman in a single room if she requires hospitalization (NICE 2016). Rarely, treatment can lead to a non-infective form of hepatitis, and liver function tests can be used to detect this (PHE 2013; Stephen & Teirstein 2013). Rifampicin can lead to orange discolouration of the urine and tears (Stephen & Teirstein 2013). Treating pregnant women with HIV for TB poses difficulties because of the combined toxicities of drug treatments, multiple side effects, high compliance requirements and potential drug interactions (Bates et al 2015).

Perinatal issues

Some babies of mothers with TB contract a congenital infection, which can range from a subclinical infection to birth defects (Bates et al 2015). Congenital TB may result from inhaling or ingesting infected amniotic fluid at birth or umbilical cord transfer; it is rare but is linked with adverse outcomes. For babies whose mothers are infected but have not received 2 weeks' treatment, prophylactic treatment with INH and pyridoxine is recommended, with a tuberculin skin test (TST) and assessment for active TB at 3 months (PHE 2013). First-line anti-TB drugs are also generally considered safe for mothers who are breastfeeding, and unless the mother has TB mastitis, the infection cannot transfer through breast milk (PHE 2013).

Activity

The Green Book (PHE 2018) recommends offering bacillus Calmette–Guerin (BCG) vaccine to people considered to be at increased risk of developing severe TB. Find out which people are considered most vulnerable and how and when the vaccine might be administered.

In particular, find out about the guidance relating to pregnancy, breastfeeding and babies who are born preterm.

Sarcoidosis

Sarcoidosis is a rare multi-system disorder which causes inflammatory granuloma (lumps) to form in the affected organ(s) (Sarcoidosis UK 2018). In pregnancy, sarcoidosis may be linked with older maternal age and smoking (Hadid et al 2015), although the precise cause is unknown (Sarcoidosis UK 2018). The lungs and skin are most commonly affected and, along with cardiac or neurological sarcoidosis, can be difficult to treat. There may be no symptoms, although some people experience a cough or dyspnoea, a rash, eye and visual symptoms and enlarged salivary glands and lymph nodes (Stephen & Teirstein 2013).

Pulmonary sarcoidosis can be diagnosed by chest X-ray or bronchoscopy. In most cases, people with pulmonary sarcoidosis have little change in respiratory function and require no treatment; any deterioration in pulmonary functioning may be treated by daily corticosteroids (Stephen & Teirstein 2013).

Sarcoidosis in pregnancy

Sarcoidosis does not appear to impair fertility in women and for most women is not a contraindication to pregnancy; pre-conception care and assessment of respiratory function can help inform women's decision-making (Vahid et al 2007). Whilst some cases of sarcoidosis improve during pregnancy, other women's respiratory function deteriorates, necessitating increased doses of corticosteroids. As pregnancy advances, women with sarcoidosis require assessments of pulmonary function: increases in circulating blood volume can impair respiration and sometimes cardiac function (Stephen & Teirstein 2013). In addition, sarcoidosis is linked with an increase in pregnancy complications such as pulmonary embolism, pre-eclampsia and eclampsia, venous thromboembolic disorders, postpartum haemorrhage and premature birth (Hadid et al 2015).

Treatment

Careful fluid management, oxygen supplementation and potentially limiting the length of labour require close involvement of a senior obstetrician and anaesthetist (Stephen & Teirstein 2013). Corticosteroids such as prednisolone can cross the placenta, and although its use is not associated with *major* congenital malformations, there appears to be a link with oral clefts, prematurity and babies who are small for gestational age; higher doses may be associated with miscarriage and perinatal death (Vahid et al 2007). Women with sarcoidosis can breastfeed as normal (Sarcoidosis UK 2018). However, prednisolone crosses into breast milk; low doses and breastfeeding 3 to 4 hours after taking the drug reduce transfer to the baby. Follow-up appointments are important since the condition can worsen a few months following birth (Vahid et al 2007).

REFLECTION ON THE TRIGGER SCENARIO

Look back on the trigger scenario.

Chantelle is 17 years old and has had asthma since she was 6 years old. Many of her close family are cigarette smokers, and she began smoking at age 14. She has had regular inhaler medication prescribed for her asthma, although she doesn't always remember to use the preventer. She is unsure about whether using her inhaler could harm her baby so has only used it on a couple of occasions, even though she has felt breathless at times. Chantelle is anxious about arranging a booking appointment, thinking that she will probably be criticized for smoking.

Chantelle's scenario is one that demonstrates a link between smoking and respiratory disease. In addition, this situation highlights the importance of midwives acknowledging that a woman's lifestyle and attitudes to healthcare provision are determined by multiple factors. Now that you are familiar with some ways in which respiratory disorders can impact on childbearing and vice versa, you should have a better understanding about how the scenario relates to the evidence. The jigsaw model will now be used to explore the trigger scenario in more depth.

Effective communication

Women value effective and consistent communication; information-sharing can build women's confidence in decision-making (National Maternity Review (NMR) 2016) and is integral to the safety and well-being of women and their babies. Chantelle's fear of being judged could have deterred her from accessing midwifery care and important information. Questions that might arise from this situation include: What physical, emotional or psychosocial factors can act as barriers to effective communication in midwifery practice and why? How can midwives and other health professionals address these barriers? How can midwives be sure that they are using the most effective method of communicating information?

Woman-centred care

It is important that women are able to choose the care that is most appropriate for their individual needs. For some women, being labelled as high or low risk limits the choices available to them (NMR 2016). In relation to Chantelle's scenario, midwives might ask the following questions: What is the purpose of using a high- or low-risk label in relation to pregnancy care? How might a high-risk label affect Chantelle's pregnancy experiences? What can midwives do to ensure that women's care is personalized and appropriate to their needs? What information is available in primary care to promote early booking with the midwife?

Using best evidence

There are greater risks of significant problems for childbearing women with pre-existing medical conditions, such as respiratory disorders (Royal College of Obstetricians and Gynaecologists (RCOG) 2016), and midwives are responsible for supporting these women in the care they are offered. Considering Chantelle's scenario, questions might include: How can midwives maintain an understanding of contemporary practice for conditions that fall outside their area of expertise? How can midwives use reflective accounts to demonstrate the currency of their knowledge? What resources are available to support women's understanding about their specific respiratory condition?

Professional and legal issues

Safety is the key priority in providing care for women and their babies. Midwives have a personal and professional accountability for ensuring that they are up to date, and their employers should provide a system of care that supports their responsibilities (RCOG 2016). Questions that arise from this scenario might include: What are the key principles of clinical governance? How might a trust's clinical governance framework support accountable midwifery practice? If women such as Chantelle choose not to follow the recommended management of their medical conditions or their pregnancy, what actions can midwives take to protect the women, themselves and their employer?

Team working

Knight and Nelson-Piercy (2017:52) recommend that to improve maternal outcomes, 'women with complex medical problems need a consultant to take a clear leadership role' In relation to women with respiratory disorders, consultants from different branches of medicine may need to collaborate. Questions that arise from the scenario might include: Which specialists might collaborate to enhance Chantelle's health during and after pregnancy? What strategies can be used to promote a cohesive approach to Chantelle's respiratory and pregnancy care? How could involving Chantelle in reviewing and adapting her PAAP impact on her own and her baby's future health?

Clinical dexterity

Women with asthma are likely to measure and record their PEF readings regularly as part of their PAAP. Midwives may be unfamiliar with the use of flow meters, the significance of the readings or how to administer asthma treatment. Questions that arise from the scenario might include: What information is documented in a PAAP that can contribute to the midwife's overall assessment of women with asthma? How can midwives differentiate between normal respiratory adaptations to pregnancy and conditions that require further investigation? What can the midwife do to gain competence and confidence in supporting women's use of asthma treatment?

Models of care

Continuity of carer is recommended to improve safety through trusting and respectful relationships between women and the professionals providing their care (NMR 2016). However, women with respiratory disorders are likely to have care from a range of specialists as well as their community midwife. Questions that arise from the scenario might include: Where might the booking appointment take place? What models of care are likely to be available for Chantelle? How can Chantelle access support and advice between appointments? In what ways can midwives promote normality for women with medical conditions?

Safe environment

Midwives are responsible for ensuring that they provide a care environment that is physically and emotionally safe for women. They are responsible for assessing the wellbeing of women and their babies throughout the childbearing period. Questions that arise from the scenario might include: How has pre-conceptual advice been addressed in the asthma clinic? What emotional factors might prevent Chantelle from accessing midwifery care? How can midwives assess whether women are using prescribed treatments appropriately? How might the use of PAAPs improve outcomes for Chantelle and her baby?

Promotes health

At least one-quarter of hospital admissions for respiratory disease are due to conditions caused by cigarette smoking (British Lung Foundation 2018). Chantelle's baby is at increased risk of developing respiratory and other problems if the people around him or her smoke. Questions that arise from the scenario might include: At what stage of Chantelle's pregnancy can the midwife make a referral for smoking cessation support? What might be the impact of involving Chantelle's family in discussions about smoking cessation? What are the other health benefits of not smoking? Who is responsible for offering Chantelle a seasonal flu vaccine? When can this be offered to pregnant women?

Further scenarios

The following scenarios enable you to consider how specific situations influence the care the midwife provides. Use the jigsaw model to explore the issues raised in the scenario.

Suraya has recently moved to the UK from Afghanistan. She is 24 weeks pregnant when she first meets her community midwife. During this appointment the midwife notes that Suraya's body mass index is 17.5 kg/m^2 and that she is tired and has a persistent cough.

Practice point

Women who are new to the UK may not understand the NHS care system and may have medical conditions that are undiagnosed or untreated. Although the midwife might have little knowledge of Suraya's previous socio-economic circumstances and health record, she should recognize that Suraya is underweight and has symptoms that could suggest a respiratory disorder.

Questions that could be asked are:
1. What can the midwife ask to get a clearer understanding of the possible causes of Suraya's current health issues?
2. What factors could hinder the midwife's ability to obtain a comprehensive history from Suraya?
3. What investigations can be ordered to confirm or rule out a diagnosis of TB?
4. What advice should be offered to Suraya to reduce the chance of transmitting TB infection to other people?
5. How might Suraya's current social circumstances affect her wellbeing, and what questions can the midwife ask to build an understanding of Suraya's needs?
6. How can Suraya's baby be protected against developing TB infection after birth?

SCENARIO 2

Rachel is 38 weeks pregnant and is generally healthy. She attends a routine antenatal appointment and explains to her community midwife that over the last few days she has been feeling increasingly breathless even when she is resting.

Practice point

Being able to differentiate between physiological and pathological causes of breathlessness is important for midwives, who are often women's first point of contact. Midwives' understanding about the possible reasons for breathlessness and their skills in assessing women's wellbeing can be crucial to women receiving appropriate care.

Questions that could be asked are:

1. What are the possible causes of breathlessness in women who are pregnant or have recently given birth? Consider physiological and pathological causes.
2. What symptoms might make the midwife suspect a pathological cause of breathlessness?
3. Which observations of the woman's condition should be recorded to assess the severity and impact of breathlessness? How and why might the clinical setting affect which assessments are performed?
4. How might midwives differentiate between breathlessness that requires urgent referral to a specialist and breathlessness that requires emergency care?
5. Where is the most appropriate place for managing acute breathlessness in a pregnant or postnatal woman?
6. How can acute respiratory disorders affect fetal wellbeing, and how can this be monitored?

Conclusion

Midwives must be confident in their understanding about normal physiological changes in respiration so that they can recognize and respond appropriately to suspected pathology. A number of respiratory disorders can affect pregnancy and vice versa; midwives are likely to be involved in providing care for women with some of these conditions. Clear and effectively communicated care planning for each stage of a woman's childbearing journey, as well as appropriate and accessible pre- and post-conceptual care, can help improve the experience and outcomes of pregnancy and childbearing for women with respiratory disorders. All professionals involved in the care of childbearing women with these conditions have a responsibility to ensure that women are provided with information and the support they need to access appropriate physical and emotional care in relation to both their respiratory disorder and their pregnancy.

Resources

Asthma UK: https://www.asthma.org.uk/advice/manage-your-asthma/pregnancy/
British Lung Foundation: https://www.blf.org.uk/
Cystic Fibrosis Trust: https://www.cysticfibrosis.org.uk/life-with-cystic-fibrosis/family-planning
Mothers and Babies: Reducing Risk through Audits and Confidential Enquiries across the UK (MBRRACE): https://www.npeu.ox.ac.uk/mbrrace-uk
Sarcoidosis UK: https://www.sarcoidosisuk.org/information-hub/about-sarcoidosis/

References

Ahluwalia, M., Hoag, J.B., Hadeh, A., et al., 2014. Cystic fibrosis and pregnancy in the modern era: a case control study. J. Cyst. Fibros. 13, 69–73. http://dx.doi.org/10.1016/j.jcf.2013.08.004.

Asthma UK, 2016. Asthma and pregnancy. Available at: https://www.asthma.org.uk/advice/manage-your-asthma/pregnancy/.

Barnett, R., 2018. Tuberculosis. Lancet 390, 351. Available at: thelancet.com.

Baston, H., Hall, J., 2018. Midwifery Essentials: Emergency Maternity Care, vol. 6. Elsevier, London.

Bates, M., Ahmed, Y., Kapta, N., et al., 2015. Perspectives on tuberculosis in pregnancy. Int. J. Infect. Dis. 32, 124–127. http://dx.doi.org/10.1016/j.ijid.2014.12.14.

Bhatia, P.K., Biyani, G., Mohammed, S., Sethi, P., 2016. Acute respiratory failure and mechanical ventilation in pregnant patient: a narrative review of literature. J. Anaesthesiol. Clin. Pharmacol. 32, 431–439. Available at: http://www.joacp.org/temp/JAnaesthClinPharmacol324431-3512132_094521.pdf.

British Lung Foundation (BLF), 2018. Lung disease in the UK – big picture statistics. Available at: https://statistics.blf.org.uk/lung-disease-uk-big-picture.

British Thoracic Society and Scottish Intercollegiate Guidelines Network, 2016. British Guideline on the management of asthma: A National Clinical Guideline. Available at: https://www.sign.ac.uk/assets/sign153.pdf.

Dyer, C., 2010. Tuberculosis. Greenwood, Oxford.

Hadid, V., Patenaude, V., Oddy, L., Abenhaim, H.A., 2015. Sarcoidosis and pregnancy: obstetrical and neonatal outcomes in a population-based cohort of 7 million births. J. Perinat. Med. 43 (2), 201–207. doi:10.1515/jpm-2014-0017.

Knight, M., Nelson-Piercy, C., on behalf of the Medical and Surgical Chapter-Writing Group, 2017. Lessons for the care of women with medical and general surgical disorders. In: Knight, M., Nair, M., Tuffnell, D., et al, on behalf of MBRRACE-UK (Eds.), Saving Lives, Improving Mothers' Care – Lessons Learned to Inform Maternity Care From the UK and Ireland Confidential Enquiries Into Maternal Deaths and Morbidity 2013–15. National Perinatal Epidemiology Unit, University of Oxford, Oxford, pp. 50–58.

Kriebs, J.M., 2015. Medical complications in pregnancy. In: King, T.L., Brucker, M.C., Kriebs, J.M., et al. (Eds.), Varney's Midwifery, fifth ed. Jones & Bartlett, Burlington, MA, pp. 773–792.

Kroon, M.A., Akkerman-Nijland, A.M., Rottier, B.L., et al., 2018. Drugs during pregnancy and breastfeeding in women diagnosed with cystic fibrosis – An update. J. Cyst. Fibros. 17, 17–25. https://doi.org/10.1016/j.jcf.2017.11.009.

Marshall, J., Baston, H., Hall, J., 2019. Midwifery Essentials. Public Health in Maternity Care. Elsevier, Edinburgh.

Mehta, N., Chen, K., Hardy, E., Powrie, R., 2015. Respiratory disease in pregnancy. Best Pract. Res. Clin. Obstet. Gynaecol. 29 (5), 598–611. https://doi.org/10.1016/j.bpobgyn.2015.04.005.

Morten, M., Collinson, A., Murphy, V.E., et al., 2018. Managing Asthma in Pregnancy (MAP) trial: FENO levels and childhood asthma. J. Allergy Clin. Immunol. doi:10.1016/j.jaci.2018.02.039. Available on-line March 8 2018.

National Consensus Standards for the Nursing Management of Cystic Fibrosis (NCSNMCF), 2016. Cystic Fibrosis: our focus. Available at: https://www.cysticfibrosis.org.uk.

National Institute for Health and Care Excellence (NICE), 2016. Tuberculosis. Available at: https://www.nice.org.uk/guidance/ng33.

National Institute for Health and Care Excellence (NICE), 2017a. Asthma: diagnosis, monitoring and chronic asthma management. Available at: https://www.nice.org.uk/guidance/ng80.

National Institute for Health and Care Excellence (NICE), 2017b. Cystic Fibrosis: diagnosis and management. Available at: https://www.nice.org.uk/guidance/ng78.

National Maternity Review, 2016. Better Births: Improving outcomes of maternity services in England. A five year forward view for maternity care. Available at: https://www.england.nhs.uk/wp-content/uploads/2016/02/national-maternity-review-report.pdf.

Preston, W., Kelly, C., 2016. Respiratory Nursing at a Glance. Wiley & Sons.

Public Health England (PHE), 2013. Pregnancy and Tuberculosis. Available at: https://assets.publishing.service.gov.uk/government/uploads/system/uploads/attachment_data/file/487319/Pregnancy_TB-Clinicians.pdf.

Public Health England, 2018. Tuberculosis. In: The Green Book. Available at: https://www.gov.uk/government/collections/immunisation-against-infectious-disease-the-green-book.

Rankin, J., 2017. Respiration. In: Rankin, J. (Ed.), Physiology in Childbearing With Anatomy and Related Biosciences, fourth ed. Elsevier, London, pp. 183–194.

Royal College of Obstetricians and Gynaecologists (RCOG), 2016. Providing Quality Care for Women: A framework for maternity service standards. Available at: https://www.rcog.org.uk/globalassets/documents/guidelines/working-party-reports/maternitystandards.pdf.

Sarcoidosis UK, 2018. Sarcoidosis and Children. Available at: https://www.sarcoidosisuk.org.

Stephen, M.J., Teirstein, A.S., 2013. Respiratory disease. In: Cohen, W., August, P. (Eds.), Management of Medical Disorders in Pregnancy, sixth ed. pp. 183–219. Available at: https://ebookcentral.proquest.com/lib/HUD/detail.action?docID=3386949.

Vahid, B., Mushlin, N., Weibel, S., 2007. Sarcoidosis in pregnancy and postpartum period. Curr. Respir. Med. Rev. 3, 79–83. https://doi.org/10.2174/157339807779941749.

CHAPTER 5

Disorders of the blood

TRIGGER SCENARIO

Charity is brought to the antenatal clinic at 34 weeks pregnant by her sister. Charity is from West Africa and has been a resident in the country for 10 years. She has had some experience of breathlessness and feeling dizzy on standing. On taking her blood pressure, the midwife notes it is 80/40 and Charity's pulse is rapid.

Introduction

Our blood supply provides important functions in the respiratory system, removing waste from the body and dealing with infection. In pregnancy it also has the extra function of supporting the growth of the baby through the placenta. Some women develop conditions during their pregnancy that affect the blood (acquired conditions), while others have hereditary conditions that may impact on pregnancy. This chapter will cover some of these circumstances, with a particular focus on anaemia.

Anaemia in pregnancy

It is a common phenomenon for women to experience a physiological drop in the iron concentration of their blood during the second trimester due to a change in plasma volume (Baston & Hall 2018:113). However, this section will focus on true anaemia, that is, non-physiological. Anaemia is a condition that is caused by a deficiency of red blood cells (RBCs) or of the quantity of haemoglobin (Hb) within them. As Hb has the role of carrying oxygen to the cells in the body, lack of them may cause some unpleasant symptoms with an impact on the woman's well-being and that of the growing fetus. Box 5.1 lists some of the potential signs and symptoms that the woman may experience.

Box 5.1 **Signs and symptoms of anaemia**

Fatigue	Breathless on exertion
Pallor of the mucous membranes	Palpitations
Headaches	Digestive upset and loss of appetite
Dizziness, fainting	Feeling cold
General weakness	Pica (craving for non-food items)

Adapted from (Bothamley & Boyle 2017:922)

Activity

Review your knowledge of the development of normal blood cells.

Review your knowledge of the blood circulation system and the role of RBCs in carrying oxygen.

What blood tests are carried out in pregnancy? What is the usual Hb result, and how would anaemia be established?

Iron-deficiency anaemia

The World Health Organization (WHO n.d. a) states that globally deficiency in iron is the most common cause of anaemia but that other deficiencies of folate, vitamin B_{12} and vitamin A may also be the reason, along with chronic inflammation conditions, infection by parasites and inherited disorders (some of which will be referred to in this chapter). It is suggested that between 24% and 49% of pregnant women populations globally have clinical anaemia (WHO 2015). With transience of populations, and adaptations to diet, it is important to recognize the potential of anaemia in pregnant women.

Activity

Review what foods provide iron, folic acid, vitamin B_{12} and vitamin A in the diet.

What advice is provided currently for all pregnant women about these foods in (or before) pregnancy?

What can be the effect of low amounts of these substances on the growing fetus?

Effect on pregnancy

For many healthy women low iron levels in the blood may not have a significant impact. However, increased requirements of iron brought on through pregnancy may lead to symptoms as highlighted in Box 5.1.

Box 5.2 **Potential complications of anaemia during pregnancy**

Complications in the mother	Complications in the infant
Lower immunity leading to increased susceptibility of infection	More likely to have iron deficiency in first 3 months of life
Less capacity for work and poor performance	Impaired psychomotor and/or mental development
Disturbance to postpartum emotions and cognition	Potential association with onset of adult diseases
Preterm labour and birth	Potential low birth weight
Placental abruption	
Peripartum blood loss	

Data from (Pavord et al 2012)

Untreated iron deficiency during pregnancy may lead to complications for the woman and her baby (Box 5.2).

At the booking appointment the midwife will establish information around the general health of the woman, which includes questions regarding her diet, previous blood loss or any existing medical conditions that could lead to anaemia. Diagnosis of anaemia is through blood tests, initially full blood count (FBC) with further tests to establish the cause of deficiency if suspected. In all pregnancies, women should be offered screening tests for anaemia in early pregnancy (National Institute for Health and Care Excellence (NICE) 2008, 2017). The normal range for Hb in pregnancy is 110 g/ml at booking and 105 g/ml at 28 weeks. It is important that there is a process for following up women who are anaemic to check compliance with medication and improving iron status.

If anaemia is identified at this time, then the midwife should establish whether a referral to a member of the medical team is required for further assessment or if treatment with oral iron may initially be sufficient. In the UK all women are also offered screening for sickle cell disease (SCD) and thalassaemia as part of the national screening programme (see https://www.gov.uk/guidance/sickle-cell-and-thalassaemia-screening-programme-overview#antenatal-screening).

Activity

Review the blood tests that are offered to all women in early pregnancy and the components of the FBC. Which tests are carried out to measure iron stores? Which women are at increased risk of iron-deficiency anaemia?

Treatment

Initial assessment by a midwife will include discussion about diet. The physiological requirements for iron for women increase threefold during pregnancy. It is therefore essential to advise women with iron deficiency how to maximize absorption. This includes an increase in the amount of iron in the diet (from red meat, poultry, fish, dried beans or dark leafy vegetables), increase of vitamin C, decrease the amount of calcium-rich foods and a decrease in the amount of tea and cereals (Pavord et al 2012). Consideration should also be made in any discussion about her social needs and whether she is unable to afford an appropriate diet or the facilities to prepare food. Lifestyle choices, such as a busy work schedule that leads to poor diet habits or increased recreational drug or alcohol consumption, may have an impact on iron stores. In addition, medical conditions, such as inflammatory bowel conditions, may interfere with toleration of diet. The midwife may advise meeting with other members of the multi-disciplinary team (MDT), such as nutrition specialists, who will support the woman and develop an appropriate dietary plan.

Iron therapy

In addition to changes in diet, women with iron deficiency will be offered iron therapy. In the UK iron is not offered as a routine to all pregnant women. Once low Hb is diagnosed, oral iron supplements will be suggested as the first line of treatment. This will usually be 100 to 200 mg daily, combined with folic acid, and will be reviewed after 2 weeks with a further blood test. Midwives should advise the woman to take these an hour before meals along with some form of vitamin C such as orange juice to increase absorption (Pavord et al 2012). In more severe situations women may be prescribed injections of iron.

Activity

Find out more about the iron preparations prescribed in your practice area. What advice should be given regarding side effects of iron supplements?

How is an intramuscular iron injection given?

If iron therapy is ineffective, further investigations will be carried out, such as the measuring of red cell parameters, serum ferritin and serum and red cell folate, in order to assess the presence of underlying conditions.

Inherited blood conditions

A range of conditions are genetically inherited, which are called *haemoglobinopathies* or *Hb disorders*, and these present particular challenges during pregnancy. Normal Hb is made up of polypeptide chains (globins) with haem molecules that contain iron. Usually they contain two α globin chains and two β chains, and the structures are determined by genetics. In haemoglobinopathies there is a mutation within these structures which may or may not cause the person to be at risk of illness. Haemoglobinopathies are autosomal-recessive inherited disorders of Hb.

> ### Activity
>
> Review the genetic transmission of haemoglobinopathies and identify the meaning of the terms *autosomal*, *recessive carrier/trait*, *zygote*, *heterozygous* and *allele*.

Fig. 5.1 shows how an infant may inherit a haemoglobinopathy from parents who both have a heterozygous genetic profile. In this situation both parents have genes that have one normal allele and one mutated allele, which leads to a 1:4 chance of a baby inheriting the condition and a 1:2 chance of being a carrier.

Globally thalassaemia and SCD are the most common genetic disorders affecting thousands in the population (WHO n.d. b). They mainly affect people with origins in hotter parts of the world. It is suggested that the genetic mutation somehow protects people from malaria (Cyrklaff et al 2011). With the transience of populations, there is potential of meeting women with these conditions in pregnancy more frequently.

Screening for haemoglobinopathy in pregnancy

Ideally women should have the opportunity for pre-conception counselling to identify those who may be at higher chance of a haemoglobinopathy (NICE 2008, 2017). Some women may already know they are carriers or have the condition and will report this, while others may be unable to do so. It is advised that all pregnant women be provided information about screening and offered a blood test for identification at booking. A family origins questionnaire (FOQ) will be used to identify

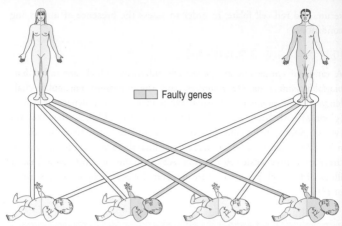

Fig. 5.1 Heterozygous inheritance. (From Myles textbook for midwives 16th ed, p 276, Fig. 13.2 'The inheritance of a haemoglobinopathy when both parents are heterozygous'.)

women at higher risk of the conditions where prevalence of the conditions are low (fewer than 1.5 fetal cases per 10,000 pregnancies) (NICE 2008, 2017). Where a woman is identified to be at greater risk or in areas of high prevalence (more than 1.5 per 10,000 pregnancies), further tests will be offered, such as high–performance liquid chromatography (HPLC).

If a woman is identified as a carrier of a condition, screening of the father of the baby will be offered, as well as counselling and tests to identify if the baby will be at risk and require further investigation (see https://www.gov.uk/government/publications/sickle-cell-and-thalassaemia-screening-care-pathway).

Sickle cell disease

SCD is so-named due to the abnormal sickle-shaped RBCs that are characteristic of the condition. It is estimated there are between 12,500 and 15,000 people with SCD in the UK (NICE 2012) and 1 in 2000 live births have the condition – about 350 babies – with another 9500 babies as carriers (NICE 2016). SCD is therefore a leading genetic condition. The condition is most frequently seen in people who are of black Caribbean, black African and black British origin, though this may affect other populations (NICE 2016). Women who carry the disease are known to have sickle cell trait (HbAS) with an adult Hb allele (A) and an abnormal allele (S). Women with the most serious condition have a genetic makeup of HbSS.

In SCD the Hb beta chain has a genetic fault which leads to damage to the RBCs. When the Hb gives up oxygen to the body tissues, the deoxygenated RBCs adopt a sickle shape and stick together. These cells become less able to move around the circulation, especially in narrow vessels. This condition leads to anaemia that requires iron therapy and may be severe enough for the person to require regular blood transfusions.

Symptoms of SCD

The symptoms will vary in severity for each person and will depend on the number of sickle cells in relation to normal RBCs present. Anaemia and fatigue will be key symptoms. If the sickle cells become stuck in the microcapillary circulation, the potential of a life-threatening event called *sickle cell crisis* may occur. Pain in relation to crisis at times will be severe and may last up to 7 days and may affect any part of the body (National Health Service (NHS) 2016). The damage caused by these blocks in the system may result in organ failure or stroke. In addition, SCD leads to an increased susceptibility to infection.

Potential complications in pregnancy

Pregnancy will add complications for a woman with SCD. Box 5.3 lists those that have been identified (Royal College of Obstetricians and Gynaecologists (RCOG) 2011). These complications lead to an increased likelihood for caesarean section, and there is a greater risk of maternal and perinatal mortality. It is therefore of importance that the midwife is caring for the woman in the context of an MDT with specialists in the condition, with early referral for any noted circumstances outside the norm.

Box 5.3 **Potential complications of SCD in pregnancy**

Spontaneous miscarriage	Pre-eclampsia and pregnancy-induced hypertension
Acute painful crisis	Infection
Fetal growth restriction	Antepartum haemorrhage
Increased premature labour	Thrombosis

From (RCOG 2011)

Awareness of potential crisis in pregnancy

It is not always possible to prevent crisis in SCD; however, it is important to recognize where pregnancy and childbirth may be a trigger. For example, preventing infection, sudden changes in temperature, dehydration, physical exertion, hypoxia and psychological stress have been listed as potential triggers (Bothamley & Boyle 2017).

Activity

Consider the list of possible triggers and think of how you would care for a woman with SCD in order to prevent a crisis.

How will you particularly provide psychological support to her and her family?

Access the RCOG (2011) guidance and find out what care is provided during a sickling crisis in your locality.

Thalassemias

Thalassemias are a group of Hb genetic disorders where the amino acid chains for either the α- or β-globin are low or misshaped, leading to short-lived RBCs and therefore lack of Hb (Modell & Darlison 2008). It mainly affects people who originate from the Mediterranean, South Asian, Southeast Asian and Middle Eastern regions. There are around 1000 people affected by thalassaemia in the UK (RCOG 2014) with many more as carriers. Globally the numbers are much higher, and again, the transience of population is leading to a likely increase within maternity services. In the UK all women are now offered screening for thalassaemia at booking. The most serious form is β-thalassaemia major (BTM). Those with known α-thalassaemia may not be affected, and usual maternity care may be continued.

Potential complications of thalassaemia

Those women with this condition are likely to have been diagnosed from childhood and therefore have lived with the condition for many years. Pre-conception advice and support should have been offered (RCOG 2014). The lack of Hb results in severe anaemia which will have required numerous blood transfusions. This will lead to an increase in the levels of iron stored in the organs of the body, which may lead to organ failure and ultimately death.

Activity

Find out about iron chelation therapy and what this involves. What drugs are used? Why would some people avoid chelation therapy? Find out about bone marrow transplantation and stem cell transplants as potential cures for thalassaemia.

If women with thalassaemia present with pregnancy, the midwife will be working as part of a specialist MDT to provide care. Specific care with respect to potential diabetes, liver function, cardiac function and thyroid function will be carried out (RCOG 2014). In addition, serial ultrasound scans will be carried out to monitor the growth and wellbeing of the baby.

Implications for midwifery practice

Midwives who provide care for women with these blood conditions should aim to provide all usual midwifery care and 'normalize' the pregnancy as much as possible within the MDT. This includes a holistic approach to care and recognizing the emotional and spiritual needs of the woman (Price et al 2007). However, the care of women with blood disorders will be delivered in partnership with a number of practitioners, and effort will need to be made to develop a supportive relationship.

Planned place of birth will likely be in a centre with neonatal facilities and specialist care available. Inclusion of the anaesthetist with planning of birth will be appropriate, as well as haematology support. For women with SCD support to give birth vaginally may be appropriate but with an aim to avoid circumstances that could trigger a crisis, such as dehydration. For women with BTM, plans for labour will be dependent on her clinical and obstetric needs at the time. Active management of the third stage will be advised (RCOG 2014).

In the postnatal period there should be an aim to avoid situations such as infection, thromboembolus and stress that could lead to a sickling crisis. Care with choice of contraception will be important, as well as genetic counselling. Midwifery care will involve psychological support around the wellbeing of the baby, especially if the baby has been admitted to a neonatal unit.

Venous thromboembolism conditions

A thrombosis is a blood clot caused by cells clumping together within the blood system. They tend to occur as a result of stasis of the blood in the veins, trauma and hypercoagulability (Merli et al 2018). These factors are known as *Virchow's triad* (Merli et al 2018). If this clot blocks a vein in the system, it may cause pain, buildup of blood flow behind it and, more seriously, damage to organs, such as in the lungs or in the brain. During pregnancy there is an increase in coagulation of the blood by about 30% (Coad & Dunstall 2011). It is stated that pregnant women in the antenatal period are about five time more at risk of a venous thromboembolism (VTE) than a non-pregnant woman (RCOG 2015) and 20 times more likely postnatally. VTE may cause serious maternal morbidity and mortality, and it remains the leading cause of direct maternal death during or up to 6 weeks after the end of pregnancy (Nair & Knight 2017), usually due to a clot lodged in the pulmonary vein.

Midwifery care

In pregnancy a thrombosis may present in the calf of the woman's leg as a deep vein thrombosis (DVT). The symptoms will include pain, swelling and inflamed skin. If suspected during pregnancy, early referral to an obstetrician should be made, who will work with other members of the MDT, such as radiologists, haematologists and physicians, to provide an appropriate plan of care. Low-molecular-weight heparin (LMWH) will be prescribed until a diagnosis by ultrasound.

Activity

Which blood tests will be carried out before administering LMWH?
Find out about LMWH, how it is administered and any side effects.
What may be the signs and symptoms of a pulmonary embolus?

In the postnatal period women are more at risk of developing a thrombosis, especially if immobile after an epidural or caesarean section. Preventive measures will be taken to avoid DVT, such as provision of

nti-embolic stockings, early mobilization, hydration and exercising of
he lower limbs to maintain circulation.

Other blood-related conditions

This chapter has focused on the main blood-related conditions that
ffect pregnancy. However, women may have or develop a vast range of
onditions, which are not feasible to describe in this chapter. This may
nclude clotting conditions such as haemophilia, von Willebrand's disease
nd platelet disorders. If a woman presents with one of these conditions,
eading about her particular condition will enhance understanding and
ecome more meaningful, as you can apply this new knowledge and ask
er about her experience living with the disease. Each woman will have
leveloped her own way of coping with the impact and managing her
ymptoms.

Activity

To find out more about these conditions locate the RCOG (2017) Green
top guideline on Management of Inherited Bleeding Disorders in
Pregnancy.

REFLECTION ON THE TRIGGER SCENARIO

Look back on the trigger scenario.

*Charity is brought to the antenatal clinic at 34 weeks pregnant by her
sister. Charity is from West Africa and has been a resident in the country
for 10 years. She has had some experience of breathlessness and feeling
dizzy on standing. On taking her blood pressure, the midwife notes it is
80/40 and Charity's pulse is rapid.*

The scenario provides a story that could take place in any clinic situation. In the chapter you will have become more aware of the potential
circumstances that could present in relation to anaemia in pregnancy.
The jigsaw model will now be used to explore the trigger scenario in
more depth.

Effective communication

Effective verbal and non-verbal communication is fundamental to the
provision of sensitive midwifery care, and essential in relation to more
complex circumstances. Questions that arise from the scenario might

include: Does Charity speak and understand English well in order for the midwife to communicate effectively, or does she require language support? What questions will the midwife ask to establish what Charity is experiencing and why? How is Charity encouraged to answer the questions? How does the midwife communicate the findings of her tests? Where and how does she document the condition, and how is this shared?

Woman-centred care

Woman-centred care ensures she is fully involved and central to the care. It should be sensitive and individualized to her needs. Questions that arise from the scenario might include: Why is Charity dizzy and her pulse fast? What are her individual health and social circumstances? How has the midwife taken these into account? How does the midwife ensure Charity is involved in the decisions for her care? How has her assessment been tailored to her individual needs? Has Charity ever experienced symptoms like these before? Does she have a family history of anaemia?

Using best evidence

To provide effective care in this situation, the midwife must use her knowledge regarding the straightforward care in pregnancy and recognize when things are more complicated. Questions that arise from the scenario might include: What potential conditions could Charity be presenting with? What is the evidence surrounding the conditions and the treatment required? What are the potential outcomes? What investigations should be carried out for assessment? Where is the best place to refer her to?

Professional and legal issues

Midwives must practise within a professional and legal framework to maintain high standards of care and protect women from potential harm. To evaluate the scenario further, you might consider the following issues: What professional and legal responsibilities are required when caring for women with a complex condition? What are the responsibilities around informed consent and sharing data? What are the responsibilities related to effective communication and documentation?

Team working

In complicated pregnancies midwives may remain the lead professional of care but also work in an MDT. Questions that arise from the scenario might include: Who else may already be involved in Charity's care? How may Charity and her family best be central to her care? Who should the midwife now refer Charity to? What is the process for contacting the medical team? How will effective team working continue during the rest of the pregnancy?

Clinical dexterity

In this circumstance clinical dexterity is required to undertake maternal observations and blood tests. The midwife will also need to monitor fetal wellbeing and growth and be able to accurately plot and record all measurements made. Questions that arise from the scenario might include: Is the midwife appropriately trained to take the tests required? Can the midwife interpret the results? Does Charity need referral elsewhere for additional tests?

Models of care

Midwives provide antenatal care in a range of different settings. How care is organized is likely to influence ongoing care for Charity and ensure effective monitoring. Questions that arise from the scenario might include: Does the midwife work in a model that provides continuity of care? What are the benefits of providing continuity of care to women with complicated conditions? If continuity is not possible, how is data shared in a confidential manner? Is there a specialist midwife who cares for women with complex needs?

Safe environment

Midwives work in a variety of locations and need to assess the risks each environment poses. Promotion of dignity and safety is paramount. Questions that arise from the scenario might include: Has Charity's comfort and dignity been maintained throughout the appointment? Does she feel safe within the environment where care is provided? Did the midwife ensure privacy and dignity was maintained at all times? Did the midwife wash her hands in between clients?

Promotes health

Antenatal care provides many opportunities to promote the health and wellbeing of both the woman and her family. This is particularly true for women with complicated conditions. Questions that arise from the scenario might include: Has the midwife explained clearly the potential seriousness of the condition? What lifestyle advice may she give Charity to help her condition in the future? Does Charity know how to get in touch with her midwife should circumstances become worse? Does she know how to contact other health professionals for support?

Further scenarios

The following scenarios enable you to consider how specific situations influence the care the midwife provides. Use the jigsaw model to explore the issues raised in the scenario.

SCENARIO 1

During a busy day in the antenatal clinic, Joanne, a 32-year-old primigravida who is 10 weeks pregnant, arrives. She has just found out that she is a healthy thalassaemia carrier and is very upset.

Practice point

In this circumstance it may be a challenge to balance the needs of Joanne, who is clearly distressed and needing time and support, and the needs of the other women who may be waiting for appointments in the clinic. Joanne will need further information, and the midwife may not have this information to hand. The main need to be met at this time will be reassurance.

Questions that could be asked are:
1. Where has Joanne received this information from? Has it been through her family or through a blood test?
2. Does the midwife have the results of the test if carried out and is she aware of the results?
3. Does the family doctor know of the results of the test?
4. Is it significant for herself and her baby that Joanne is a carrier of thalassaemia?
5. Has an FOQ been completed?
6. Has the father of the baby been tested for thalassaemia?
7. Why would this be significant?
8. How may Joanne be reassured at this time?

SCENARIO 2

Sammi, a community midwife, receives a call from Carole, a 42-year-old woman who had her first baby 4 days ago by caesarean section. Carole came from hospital yesterday and is experiencing a dull ache in the back of her left calf when she walks.

This scenario illustrates the increasing numbers of women who are giving birth at a later age and also the early days at which women are transferred home from hospital following surgery. Midwives in the community therefore need to deal with more complicated circumstances.

Questions that could be asked are:

1. What could be the diagnosis in this situation? What assessment will Sammi need to make?
2. Why would a more mature woman who has given birth be more at risk of this diagnosis?
3. What are the risk factors in this scenario that may lead to this complication?
4. What are the risks to Carole?
5. Which member of the MDT will Sammi refer her to?
6. What tests may be carried out?
7. What treatment may be required?
8. If Carole is readmitted to the hospital, what will happen to her baby?

Conclusion

Anaemia and more complicated blood conditions are of global concern and may cause serious morbidity to the mother. As there is continued global transience of populations, midwives need to have an understanding and knowledge of the conditions and how to screen for them in order to advise and support women in their care. Appropriate referral should also be made to ensure the woman provides the best and safest care in the multi-disciplinary environment.

Resources

ARC (Antenatal results and choices) https://www.arc-uk.org/tests-explained/sickle-cell-and-thalassaemia

Public Health Education *Sickle cell and thalassaemia screening: education and training* https://www.gov.uk/guidance/sickle-cell-and-thalassaemia-screening-education-and-training

Sickle cell and thalassaemia support project http://www.sctsp.org.uk/home https://www.rcog.org.uk/en/guidelines-research-services/guidelines/gtg66/

Sickle Cell Disease in Pregnancy, Management of (Green-top Guideline No. 61) Green top guideline (RCOG) https://www.rcog.org.uk/en/guidelines-research-services/guidelines/gtg61/

Thalassaemia in Pregnancy, Management of Beta (Green-top 66) Green top guideline (RCOG)

References

Baston, H., Hall, J., 2018. Midwifery Essentials: Antenatal, second ed. Elsevier, Oxford.

Bothamley, J., Boyle, M., 2017. Hypertensive and medical disorders in pregnancy. In: MacDonald, S., Johnson, G. (Eds.), Mayes' Midwifery, fifteenth ed. Elsevier, Oxford.

Coad, J., Dunstall, M., 2011. Anatomy and Physiology for Midwives, third ed. Churchill Livingstone, Edinburgh.

Cyrklaff, M., Sanchez, C.P., Kilian, N., et al., 2011. Hemoglobins S and C interfere with actin remodeling in *Plasmodium falciparum*–infected erythrocytes. Science 334 (6060), 1283–1286. doi:10.1126/science.1213775.

Merli, G., Eraso, L.H., Galanis, T., Ouma, G., 2018. Pulmonary embolism. BMJ Best Practice https://bestpractice.bmj.com/topics/en-gb/116.

Modell, B., Darlison, M., 2008. Global epidemiology of haemoglobin disorders and derived service indicators. Bull. World Health Organ. 86 (6), 417–496. http://www.who.int/bulletin/volumes/86/6/06-036673/en/.

Nair, M., Knight, M., 2017. Surveillance and Epidemiology. In: Knight, M., Nair, M., Tuffnell, D., et al. on behalf of MBRRACE-UK (Eds.), Saving Lives, Improving Mothers' Care – Lessons Learned to Inform Maternity Care From the UK and Ireland Confidential Enquiries Into Maternal Deaths and Morbidity 2013–15. National Perinatal Epidemiology Unit, University of Oxford, Oxford.

NHS, 2016. *Sickle Cell Disease.* https://www.nhs.uk/conditions/sickle-cell-disease/.

NICE, 2008. 2017. *Antenatal Care for uncomplicated pregnancies clinical guideline.* https://www.nice.org.uk/guidance/cg62.

NICE, 2012. *Sickle cell disease: managing acute painful episodes in hospital.* https://www.nice.org.uk/guidance/cg143/chapter/Introduction.

NICE CKS, 2016. Sickle cell disease. https://cks.nice.org.uk/sickle-cell-disease#!backgroundsub:1.

Pavord, S., Myers, B., Robinson, S., et al. on behalf of the British Committee for Standards in Haematology, 2012. UK guidelines on the management of iron deficiency in pregnancy. Br. J. Haematol. 156, 588–600. doi:10.1111/j.1365-2141.2011.09012.x.

Price, S., Lake, M., Breen, G., et al., 2007. The spiritual experience of high-risk pregnancy. J. Obstet. Gynecol. Neonatal Nurs. 36, 63–70. doi:10.1111/j.1552-6909.2006.00110.x.

RCOG, 2011. Management of Sickle Cell Disease in pregnancy (Green-top Guideline No. 61). https://www.rcog.org.uk/globalassets/documents/guidelines/gtg_61.pdf.

RCOG, 2014. Management of Beta Thalassaemia in pregnancy (Green-top Guideline No 64). https://www.rcog.org.uk/globalassets/documents/guidelines/gtg_66_thalassaemia.pdf.

RCOG, 2015. Thromboembolic Disease in pregnancy and puerperium: Acute management (Green top guideline No 37b). https://www.rcog.org.uk/globalassets/documents/guidelines/gtg-37b.pdf.

RCOG, 2017. Management of Inherited Bleeding Disorders in Pregnancy (Green-top Guideline No. 71). https://www.rcog.org.uk/en/guidelines-research-services/guidelines/gtg71/.

WHO, undated a. *Anaemia*. http://www.who.int/topics/anaemia/en/.

WHO, undated b. *Genes and human disease*. http://www.who.int/genomics/public/geneticdiseases/en/index2.html.

WHO, 2015. The Global Prevalence of Anaemia in 2011. World Health Organization, Geneva. http://apps.who.int/iris/bitstream/handle/10665/177094/9789241564960_eng.pdf?sequence=1.

CHAPTER 6

Digestive conditions

TRIGGER SCENARIO

Verity goes to the clinic waiting room and notices Priya, pregnant with her first baby, sitting there wriggling in her seat and scratching the palms of her hands. She invites Priya into her room for her 28-week appointment. Priya explains that she has started to have terrible itching of her skin all over her body, but it is much worse on the palms of her hands and her feet, and especially at night.

Introduction

Women may enter pregnancy with digestive conditions or may develop conditions during pregnancy. Most digestive conditions do not affect the outcome of pregnancy, but some complications may occur. For example, nausea and vomiting is a common aspect of early pregnancy, but severe vomiting, or hyperemesis gravidarum, may result in the woman needing hospital care. During the antenatal booking appointment, the woman may share information regarding her medical history such as an inflammatory bowel condition or a previous infection or cancer that may impact on her wellbeing during pregnancy. Usually she will be under the care of a medical team already, and it will be important for the midwife to work with the multi-disciplinary team (MDT) to provide relevant care. For further discussion regarding care for women with cancer, see Chapter 2, and for eating disorders, see Volume 7, Chapter 10 in the *Midwifery Essentials* series.

The aim of this chapter will be to explore the circumstances of digestive conditions in pregnancy and to discuss relevant midwifery care.

Physiology of the digestive system in pregnancy

The physical and hormonal changes that take place during pregnancy have a physiological effect on the woman's digestive system. For example, the changing hormones may impact on feelings of hunger and thirst (Coad & Dunstall 2011). These effects will be individual to the woman in the early stages and throughout pregnancy, with some experiencing changes in taste, nausea with or without vomiting, heartburn and constipation (for a summary table see Baston & Hall 2018:55). Increased levels of progesterone in pregnancy lead to reduced gastric motility and muscle tone (Rankin 2017).

Review the digestive system. Consider what happens to a woman's digestive system as a result of the normal physiological changes in pregnancy.

How would you differentiate between normal nausea and vomiting in pregnancy and (a) hyperemesis gravidarum or (b) gastroenteritis?

It is important to understand how the normal physiology may cause digestive symptoms during pregnancy that may lead to the woman seeking midwifery advice. It is also important to appreciate when these symptoms are excessive and do not follow a usual pattern. In these circumstances referral to a member of the MDT will be appropriate for further investigation or treatment. Table 6.1 lists some conditions that may present during pregnancy with the potential complications that may arise. Benign or cancerous tumours may develop or be present in any part of the digestive tract, and it is essential to refer the woman for medical review if she experiences persistent or unusual symptoms.

Gallbladder

The gallbladder is a storage organ for bile for when the body requires it to aid in digestion of fat. The impact of increased development of bile along with reduced motility of the bile duct can lead to the development of gallstones. The number of people with gallstones globally is increasing (Achalovschi & Lammert 2018). Gallbladder disease is more likely in women over the age of 40 (Wang & Portincasa 2017). With the increasing older demographic of women becoming pregnant, it is likely more gallbladder conditions will arise in pregnancy.

Review the physiological function of the gallbladder. Find out how this function is altered during pregnancy and why.

How does bile change, and what effect can this have?

Table 6.1: **Digestive conditions in pregnancy**

Location	Condition	Reason develops in pregnancy	Complications
Mouth	Stomatitis	Viral, fungal, non-infective allergic reactions	
Tongue	Inflammation	Associated with anaemia	
Salivary gland (parotid)	Hyperemesis/difficulty in swallowing	Rising level of human chorionic gonadotrophin, progesterone Associated with dry mouth	
Pharynx	Dyspepsia	Relaxation of sphincter (progesterone)	
Oesophagus	Dyspepsia (heartburn) Gastro-oesophageal reflux disease Oesophagitis	Relaxation of sphincter (progesterone) Repeated reflux/heartburn	Oesophageal ulcers
Diaphragm	Hiatus hernia	Associated with obesity and weak diaphragmatic sphincter	Strangulated hernia
Liver	HELLP/hepatitis Tumours Obstetric Cholestasis/intra-hepatitis	High blood pressure/infection/obstructions	Pruritus (increased bile salts) May lead to serious pregnancy complications for mother and or baby (tumour)
Stomach	Gastritis/gastric ulcers	Inflammation of the lining, acute or chronic Slow emptying Slight reduction in gastric secretions	Tumour
Gall bladder	Cholecystitis Cholelithiasis Choledocholithiasis	Obstruction/gallstones	Tumour
Pancreas	Pancreatitis: acute/chronic	Obstruction/alcohol abuse Development of gestational diabetes	Tumour

Table 6.1: **Digestive conditions in pregnancy** *(Continued)*

Location	Condition	Reason develops in pregnancy	Complications
Duodenum/ jejunum	Coeliac/ulcers	Reduced motility	Infection Infertility Autoimmune disease (increased risk) Haematological disorders Dermatitis Herpetiformis Tumour
Colon transverse, ascending, descending and sigmoid	Crohn's, ulcerative colitis, diverticulitis, appendicitis	Chronic inflammatory/ small pouch	Vaginal candidiasis Dyspareunia Hernia from excessive vomiting Obstruction to ileostomy/ colostomy Tumour
Ileum/ caecum	Crohn's, ulcerative colitis	Reduced motility	Tumour
Rectum	Constipation Haemorrhoids Anal sphincter injury	Reduced motility Previous pregnancy injury	Tumour

Adapted from (Davis 2009)

Pregnancy does not lead to major alterations within the liver during normal pregnancy; however, there are some changes in the functions. There can be an increase in the activity of serum alkaline phosphatase, probably due to the increased placental alkaline phosphatase isoenzymes. As a result, there will usually be a decrease in the ratio of albumin to globulin in pregnancy.

Review the anatomy and physiology of the liver. Review the physiological function of the pancreas and its role in digestion.

Find out about the role of the pancreas in relation to gestational diabetes (see Chapter 10).

Intrahepatic cholestasis

Intrahepatic or obstetric cholestasis of pregnancy is a condition where there is a buildup of bile salts that leads to pruritus (itching) without a rash and abnormal liver function tests (LFTs) (Royal College of Obstetricians and Gynaecologists (RCOG) 2011). Though in the UK it is a rare condition overall (about 7 in 1000 women in the main population), it is more common in women from Indian Asian or Pakistani Asian populations (1.5%), and globally is more common in other populations (RCOG 2011). As such, there may be genetic or environmental causes, as well as a relationship with hormonal activity (Geenes et al 2016). Women may present with symptoms of generalized itching, often commencing on the palms of the hands and the soles of the feet (Geenes et al 2016). It is also more common at night, leading to lack of sleep and subsequent fatigue. Other symptoms may be dark urine, pale stools, pain and jaundice in more severe conditions.

Though the impact on the woman is severe discomfort, it is not usually life threatening. However, the risk to the unborn fetus is more concerning, with an increased incidence of preterm birth and stillbirth (RCOG 2011).

Activity

Review the biliary system and consider why there may be symptoms of dark urine, pale stools and jaundice.

Treatment of cholestasis

If a woman presents with pruritus in pregnancy to the midwife, a careful history should be taken of the development of the condition in order to exclude other liver conditions. Referral will be made to the obstetric team for assessment of liver function and assessment of the wellbeing of the fetus. Ultrasound scans to exclude other pathology of the liver may be carried out. A balance will need to be taken for the optimum time of safety for the fetus, and therefore regular surveillance, usually weekly LFTs, will be offered until the time is felt to be the best time for birth (RCOG 2011). It is likely that a planned induction of labour and birth in a hospital unit, including active management to prevent excessive blood loss due to poor absorption of vitamin K, will be offered (RCOG 2011).

A midwife's care will involve vigilance around preterm birth and altered patterns of fetal movements. Calamine lotion or similar is recommended for the treatment of the itching, as it may provide some relief. Keeping cool, keeping nails short and wearing cotton gloves at night to prevent excessive damage to the skin though scratching at night may assist. There is no known treatment to prevent it; however, the use of ursodeoxycholic acid (UDCA) may reduce the itching and bile salts and improve outcomes for the fetus, but more research is required (RCOG 2011). In circumstances where the woman's prothrombin time is prolonged, vitamin K may be offered prior to labour in doses of 5 to 10 mg daily.

Activity

Read your local guidance on care of women with cholestasis. How will her condition be monitored?

Find out what treatment is offered to women in your location. When should induction of labour be considered? How will her labour be monitored?

Review the action of vitamin K in the body in relation to clotting.

Significantly, the midwife will need to provide psychological support to the woman, as the condition is distressing and will lead to fatigue. Reassurance that the condition will resolve following the birth of the baby should be given.

Bowel conditions

In pregnancy the presence of progesterone impacts on the smooth muscle of the gut, which leads to slower transit time of the contents, resulting in increased absorption of water and nutrients (Coad & Dunstall 2011). While this leads to an increased potential of constipation, this is of more significance for those who present in pregnancy with long-term bowel conditions. It is suggested that around 10% to 20% of the population experiences irritable bowel syndrome (IBS) – it is more common in the 20- to 30-year-old age group and twice as likely to be women than men (National Institute for Health and Care Excellence (NICE) 2008, 2017). This is clearly relevant for the pregnant population. Inflammatory bowel conditions, such as ulcerative colitis (UC) and Crohn's disease, tend to develop in young adults (Kapoor et al 2016).

Table 6.1 has listed a number of bowel conditions, but some, such as gastro-oesophageal conditions, are rare and usually not seen in women under the age of 40. These should be considered where minor disorders are prolonged or worsen in pregnancy and in those who are older than

40. Other conditions, such as haemorrhoids, are common, and complications such as strangulation and thrombosis are rare. Treatment tends to be conservative in pregnancy, but investigations should be considered where symptoms are prolonged or severe.

Irritable bowel syndrome

IBS is a chronic disorder that leads to disturbances in the bowel. It usually leads to abdominal pain with an altered bowel habit accompanied by bloating (NICE 2008, 2017). It is often only diagnosed after excluding other conditions (Robson & Waugh 2013). As pregnancy has a known impact on the bowel, leading to increased constipation, symptoms of IBS may become more troublesome.

Activity

Review the physiological reasons for constipation in pregnancy. What advice is given to women to prevent and relieve constipation in pregnancy?

Locate a copy of the Bristol stool chart and consider how this may be used to help discussion around constipation.

Women who have long-term IBS will be aware of known dietary triggers and should aim to avoid these. Maintenance of adequate fluid intake and bulking agents to relieve any constipation should be considered in consultation with the woman and members of the MDT. NICE guidance (2008, 2017) recommends a variety of dietary adaptations, including at least eight glasses or cups of clear liquid a day; restriction of tea, coffee, alcohol and fizzy drinks; and less wholemeal and high-fibre foods and use of oats instead of bran.

For women who have more serious IBS who have an *ileostomy* (small bowel diversion to open onto the abdominal surface), awareness should be made of complications with the *stoma* (opening of the bowel) in the second trimester as the uterus enlarges. Complaints of abdominal pain, which may be a sign of obstruction of the ileostomy, should be taken seriously with prompt referral for medical assessment.

Crohn's disease

In Europe the incidence of Crohn's disease is 0.3 to 12.7 per 100,000 (Kapoor et al 2016). It is a chronic inflammatory disease of the lining of the alimentary and digestive system. It is not known why this occurs, though there may be genetic factors; environmental factors such as smoking, medication, psychological factors or infection; and the gut immune system (Kapoor et al 2016). It is usually distributed irregularly, with some areas of normal bowel lining in between the affected areas. A woman may have remission at times without symptoms, but in relapse, inflammation may lead to a range of different symptoms. These include diarrhoea, abdominal pain, fever, fatigue and weight loss (Robson & Waugh 2013). In addition, women may experience sore mouths and eyes, and there is an association with arthritis. In severe cases, a woman may have an ileostomy or colostomy (large bowel diversion to open onto the abdominal surface) in place. There is currently no known cure, and the aim will be to reduce symptoms and to maintain remission (NICE 2012, 2016).

Activity

Find out the effect of active Crohn's disease on the reproductive system and fertility.

Review the physiological effect of pregnancy on the blood system. Consider the effect of major diarrhoea on the nutritional status of women who become pregnant with Crohn's disease and the impact on pregnancy.

During pregnancy, joint care should be provided with physicians and across the MDT. Control of the disease is important, as active disease is associated with miscarriage, fetal intrauterine growth restriction (IUGR) and premature birth (Robson & Waugh 2013), and drug therapy will usually be maintained. Specific monitoring for anaemia will be important due to the deficiency in the diet of iron, folate or vitamin B_{12}.

Activity

Find out what medication is currently used to control Crohn's disease. Is this safe in pregnancy?

Ulcerative colitis

In contrast to Crohn's disease UC is a chronic autoimmune disease of the bowel causing mucosal inflammation. It may only be rectal disease but can extend into the sigmoid colon and the whole digestive system. In Europe, the annual incidence of UC ranges from 0.6 to 24.3 per 100,000 (Kapoor et al 2016) and tends to develop in the 15- to 35-year-old age group (Robson & Waugh 2013). It is thought UC may be caused by genetic or environmental factors and, for some reason, smoking appears to provide a protective effect (Robson & Waugh 2013). Symptoms are similar to those with Crohn's but are marked by visible blood in the stool and the passage of mucus (Kapoor et al 2016).

Activity

Find out what pre-conception assessment may be advised prior to pregnancy for women with UC.

Find out what medication is usually prescribed for the condition.

During pregnancy joint care should be provided across the MDT with effective communication and information-sharing to ensure the woman receives appropriate treatment (NICE 2013). Her medication will be discussed with her to present the risks and benefits of maintaining the drugs or stopping them and the chances of relapse (NICE 2013). Care will usually be maintained in the community, though there are risks of haemorrhage, IUGR and premature birth (Robson & Waugh 2103).

Monitoring of weight will usually be required, and a dietician may be required to support the woman in creating a diet plan and preventing malnourishment (Robson & Waugh 2013). She should be encouraged to monitor her stools for blood, consistency, frequency and condition (Robson & Waugh 2103). During any admission to hospital, she should be situated in a room near a toilet.

There is evidence to suggest a link between UC and mood disorder (Cawthorpe 2015). Women with UC will need support and empathy, as the condition may be debilitating and may have an impact on her self-esteem.

Coeliac disease

Coeliac disease is an inflammatory condition of the bowel mucosa induced by gluten in the diet. It appears to have immune, genetic and environmental predisposing factors (Butler et al 2011). It can cause atrophy of the intestinal villi, and damage in the small bowel leads to malabsorption (Robson & Waugh 2013). Population studies suggest around 1 in 100 people in the UK are affected by the disease (NICE 2015).

Activity

Find out what foodstuffs contain gluten.

How do you arrange a gluten-free diet to be available for women in your unit?

Box 6.1 **Coeliac disease symptoms (NICE 2015)**

Gastrointestinal	Non-gastrointestinal
Indigestion	Fatigue
Diarrhoea	Dermatitis herpetiformis
Abdominal Pain	Anaemia
Bloating	Osteoporosis
Distension	Reproductive problems
Constipation	Neuropathy
	Ataxia
	Delayed puberty

The symptoms experienced are varied. Box 6.1 lists the potential symptoms experienced with the disease (NICE 2015). It suggests that for some, the symptoms are more severe than for others.

The condition is managed through a gluten-free diet. During pregnancy the aid of a dietician may be required to ensure the wellbeing of the woman and her baby and to prevent malnutrition. In particular, women with coeliac disease should take a higher dose of folic acid, preferably pre-conception and in early pregnancy, to prevent neural tube defects in the growing baby. Uncontrolled coeliac disease leads to a higher risk of miscarriage and is associated with low birth weight, IUGR and preterm birth (Butler et al 2011). Women with coeliac disease should receive consultant-led care.

Activity

Find out what neural tube defects are in babies, when these develop and the effect of folic acid.

Locate and read the original study related to the use of folic acid in pregnancy (Medical Research Council Vitamin Study 1991). What food-stuffs are a good source of folic acid?

As with other digestive system conditions, malabsorption of iron may lead to anaemia, and careful screening should be carried out (Robson & Waugh 2013).

Provision of holistic midwifery care

A woman with a known condition may have already met with specialists in order to ensure she is as well as she can be for pregnancy. She may have a clear understanding of how her condition might affect her pregnancy or how her pregnancy might affect her condition. The midwife should listen carefully to the woman, as she is likely to be 'expert' in her needs. For women with known conditions of the digestive system, the midwife will need to be aware of the impact of the condition on her physically and emotionally, as well as recognize her needs for support and that of her family. She will need to communicate effectively and take an accurate booking history and assessment to establish the nature of the condition and how it impacts on her daily life. Careful listening to the woman's concerns will be essential, as an alteration in symptoms may indicate that complications have developed (see Table 6.1).

An accurate history of any medication should be recorded. Calculation of the body mass index and weight of the woman may be appropriate in early pregnancy to provide a baseline for any changes. Establishing her dietary needs will be necessary with referral to a dietician as required.

The midwife will need to work in a referral and liaison role, which means working effectively with the multi-professional team (NMC 2015).

Activity

Find out in your locality how a community-based midwife refers care of a woman to:

A general practitioner: obstetrician: A specialist doctor in the digestive system: dietician.

After referral, how does a community-based midwife ensure she still provides midwifery care for the woman?

Medication requirements will be individual for each woman and the type of condition. Any treatment needs to be balanced with the needs of the developing fetus and the woman's reaction to pregnancy. Drugs taken during active disease in the first trimester may affect the developing fetus; therefore liaison with specialist medical practitioners is essential.

Activity

Find out what medicines are used in your locality for each of the conditions in Table 6.1.

Establish how these are administrated and the potential side effects, including the impact on the baby and use in breastfeeding

Diagnosis of a digestive disorder in pregnancy

Pregnant women who develop a medical condition may experience a number of emotions such as apprehension, anxiety, fear, denial and even confusion regarding the advice available. Pain may increase stress levels. Needing to spend time in hospital may be necessary, which may lead to anxiety for a woman and her family who is having their second baby or who has other family dependents at home. The woman may also express concern for her fetus/baby. A condition such as acute appendicitis may occasionally mean giving birth to a preterm baby. The midwife will then have to care for a pre- and post-operative woman concerned about her baby.

Midwives may also need to gain the support of other members of the MDT in order to care for women with unfamiliar conditions. For example, this may be wound care nurses or colostomy and ileostomy nurses who can give advice on bags to use in pregnancy and the postnatal period (NICE 2008, 2017).

Surgery for digestive conditions

Generally, the decision regarding surgery for conditions in pregnancy should be weighed against the risk to the woman or the fetus if surgery is not carried out (Skubic & Salim 2017). Gallbladder disease and appendicitis tend to be the two most common reasons for surgery, but this will normally be a last resort should conservative management be ineffective. A laparoscopic method is recommended to avoid injury to the uterus and the fetus and appears to be mainly safe (Nasioudis et al 2016). It is important to monitor the woman carefully following surgery as preterm labour may be triggered (Robson & Waugh 2013).

Activity

Consult local guidelines on caring for women with digestive disorders. Find out how to care for a woman who has surgery for these conditions during or after pregnancy.

Implications for labour

Supportive care for women with medical conditions is essential. At all times appropriate monitoring of the woman and fetus should be undertaken during labour according to the condition. Continuous electronic monitoring may be appropriate in some circumstances, such as obstetric cholestasis, but not in all situations. For most conditions, such as UC and Crohn's, there is no reason that care in labour may not be straightforward, and in the absence of complications, the woman will progress in labour with care by the midwife.

Discussion with the woman about avoiding a prolonged second stage or straining in labour may have taken place as part of the intrapartum plans for conditions such as hiatus hernia, haemorrhoids and UC. Where the condition may lead to concerns about anaemia, a full blood count should be carried out to check her haemoglobin status to prepare for and be aware of excessive blood loss during the third stage. Prevention of dehydration during labour will also be essential.

Activity

Consider how you would care for a woman who has a known digestive condition in labour.

Find out the protocol for caring for women with intrahepatic cholestasis in your location.

Postnatal implications

The majority of women with digestive conditions will have a physiologically normal postnatal period and will require midwifery-based care. For some, where treatments have been commenced prior to or during pregnancy, such as changes in diet, these should continue following birth. Specialist medical support may be required to adjust medications or diets, as there may be physical adjustment as the impact of hormonal changes takes place. Good hygiene to prevent infection should be maintained and awareness of the potential for faecal incontinence.

Psychological care will be required, as some women will be adjusting to a new diagnosis, as well as coping with being a new parent. Midwives should also be aware of those women experiencing fatigue following birth, as well as potential anaemia, as they may require increased support with caring for the baby.

Infant feeding should be discussed early, as drugs used in pregnancy may have an effect on the baby; advice should be sought for these women and their partners. Breastfeeding should be promoted where it is believed to be protective in the delay of the condition for the child (coeliac disease). Babies may need monitoring for the clinical signs of immunosuppressants (UC).

Look back on the trigger scenario.

Verity goes to the clinic waiting room and notices Priya, pregnant with her first baby, sitting there wriggling in her seat and scratching the palms of her hands. She invites Priya into her room for her 28-week appointment. Priya explains that she has started to have terrible itching of her skin all over her body, but it is much worse on the palms of her hands and her feet, and especially at night.

The scenario provides a story that could take place in any clinic situation. Now that you are familiar with the potential circumstances that could present in relation to digestive medical conditions, you may have some insight into the condition presented and the evidence surrounding care. The jigsaw model will now be used to explore the trigger scenario in more depth.

Effective communication

The use of effective verbal and non-verbal communication is fundamental to the provision of sensitive midwifery care. Observation and listening are also important skills. Questions that arise from the scenario might include: How did Verity make Priya feel welcome into the room? What questions were asked and in what way? How did Verity encourage Priya to answer the questions? Does Priya communicate well in the English language, or does she require translation support? How does Verity communicate what condition she was observing? Where and how does she document the condition, and how is this shared?

Woman-centred care

In order to ensure a woman is central to her care, the midwife needs to be sensitive and ensure care is individualized to her needs. This entails involving the woman in her care and providing appropriate information so that she can make informed choices. Questions that arise from the scenario might include: Why is Priya experiencing itching? What are her individual circumstances? Has Verity found out what her circumstances are? How is Priya involved in the decision making around her care? Is the assessment of her pregnancy at this time tailored to her individual needs?

Using best evidence

To provide effective care in this situation, the midwife must use her knowledge regarding the straightforward care in pregnancy and recognize where things are more complicated. Questions that arise from the scenario might include: What is the condition that Priya could be presenting with? What is the evidence surrounding the condition and the treatment required? What are the potential outcomes? Where should Priya be referred for assessment?

Professional and legal issues

Midwives must practise within a professional and legal framework to maintain high standards of care and protect women from potential harm. To evaluate the scenario further, you might consider the following issues: What professional and legal responsibilities are required when caring for women with a complex condition? What are the responsibilities around informed consent and sharing data? What are the responsibilities related to effective communication and documentation?

Team working

In complicated pregnancies midwives may remain the lead professional of care but work as well in an MDT. Questions that arise from the scenario might include: Who else may already be involved in Priya's care? Who should Priya now be referred to, and what is the process for contacting the medical team? How will effective team working continue during the rest of the pregnancy? How may Priya and her family best be central to her care?

Clinical dexterity

Performing observational and clinical tasks during Priya's care will help her have confidence in the skill and knowledge of her midwife. For example, Priya may require close monitoring of her liver function for the rest of her pregnancy, and it is likely that multiple blood tests may be required. Questions that arise from the scenario might include: Is the midwife appropriately trained to take the bloods required? Does Verity have sufficient understanding of the blood tests to gain informed consent? Where will the results of the blood tests go, and who will be informed of the results?

Models of care

Midwives provide antenatal care in a range of settings. How care is organized is likely to influence ongoing care for Priya and effective monitoring. Questions that arise from the scenario might include: Does Verity work in a model that provides continuity of care? What are the benefits of providing continuity to women with complicated conditions? If continuity is not possible, how are data shared in a confidential manner?

Safe environment

Midwives work in a variety of locations and need to assess the risks each environment poses. Promotion of dignity and safety is paramount. Questions that arise from the scenario might include: Has the woman's comfort and dignity been maintained throughout the appointment? Does she feel safe within the environment? Did the midwife wash her hands in between clients? How will the needle and any clinical waste be safely disposed of?

Promotes health

Antenatal care provides many opportunities to promote the health and wellbeing of both the woman and her family. This is particularly true for women with complicated conditions. Questions that arise from the scenario might include: Has Verity explained clearly the potential seriousness of the condition? Does Priya know how to get in touch with her midwife should circumstances become worse? Does she know how to contact other health professionals for support?

Further scenarios

The following scenarios enable you to consider how specific situations influence the care the midwife provides. Use the jigsaw model to explore the issues raised in the scenario.

SCENARIO 1

Jodie is a 20-year-old woman with long-term UC who presents in the clinic at 14 weeks with an unexpected pregnancy.

Practice point

In these circumstances it is more usual for a woman to have discussed pregnancy pre-conception with the medical team and ensured she is in optimum health prior to pregnancy. In this scenario there is a potential that Jodie may be less well and require extra support.

Questions that could be asked are:
1. Is Jodie experiencing particular complications with UC at this time?
2. Is her condition well managed at this time?
3. Does she require urgent referral for medical assessment, and who should she be referred to?
4. What investigations may be required?
5. What psychological support may be required?
6. What social support does Jodie have?
7. How may the wellbeing of Jodie and the baby be assessed?

SCENARIO 2

Emily contacts her midwife 3 days following an emergency caesarean birth after a long labour and attempted forceps delivery prior to this. She says she has been unable to open her bowels and when she tries it feels 'very swollen down there and painful to sit on'.

Practice point

This scenario highlights that complicated labours and births may lead to potential difficulties with the digestive system in the postnatal period. Often women are transferred home after operative birth after 24 hours, and the complications that arise are met by the community-based teams. Being prepared to meet these needs and offer appropriate effective care is paramount.

Questions that could be asked are:
1. What is the potential cause of the pain and discomfort Emily is experiencing?
2. What will be the actions of the midwife?
3. How may Emily be helped to open her bowels?
4. Is there any practical advice to ease the pain and discomfort she is experiencing?
5. Is there any medication she could be provided to help?
6. What will be done if this situation does not improve or becomes worse?

Conclusion

Women with known, or who develop, digestive conditions during pregnancy have different needs and responses to the conditions. The midwife has to clearly use many skills to properly assess and plan the individual care that is required. Monitoring gastrointestinal function is central to the care of these women, alongside essential health promotion and health education about diet.

The midwife needs to listen to the woman carefully and support and encourage her to have an awareness of any changes to her condition that occur during pregnancy and childbirth. Care should be individualized and woman-centred, and factors that warrant further investigation should be looked for and documented, as diagnosis of the conditions is not always easy.

Resources

British Liver Trust https://www.britishlivertrust.org.uk/liver-information/liver-conditions/icp/

Coeliac UK https://www.coeliac.org.uk/coeliac-disease/

Crohn's and Colitis UK https://www.crohnsandcolitis.org.uk/about-us

Robson SE and Waugh J (2008). *Medical Disorders in Pregnancy: A Manual for Midwives*, Blackwell Publishing.

References

Achalovschi, M., Lammert, F., 2018. The Growing Global Burden of Gallstone Disease World Gastroenterology association. http://www.worldgastroenterology.org/publications/e-wgn/e-wgn-expert-point-of-view-articles-collection/the-growing-global-burden-of-gallstone-disease.

Baston, H., Hall, J., 2018. Midwifery Essentials, vol. 2. Antenatal 2e. Elsevier, Oxford.

Butler, M.M., Kenny, L.C., McCarthy, F.P., 2011. Coeliac disease and pregnancy outcomes. Obstet. Med. 4 (3), 95–98.

Cawthorpe, D., 2015. Temporal comorbidity of mental disorder and ulcerative colitis. Perm. J. 19 (1), 52–57.

Coad, J., Dunstall, M., 2011. Anatomy and Physiology for Midwives. Churchill Livingstone, Edinburgh.

Davis, S., 2009. Digestive conditions in pregnancy. Pract. Midwife 12 (1), 32–38.

Geenes, V., Williamson, C., Chappell, L.C., 2016. Intrahepatic cholestasis of pregnancy. The Obstetrician & Gynaecologist 18, 273–281. doi:10.1111/tog.12308.

Kapoor, D., Teahon, K., Wallace, S.V.F., 2016. Inflammatory bowel disease in pregnancy. The Obstetrician & Gynaecologist 18, 205–212. 10.1111/tog.12271.

Medical Research Council Vitamin Study Research Group, 1991. Prevention of neural tube defects: results of the Medical Research Council Vitamin Study. Lancet 338 (8760), 131–198.

Nasioudis, D., Tsilimigras, D., Economopoulos, K.P., 2016. Laparoscopic cholecystectomy during pregnancy: a systematic review of 590 patients international. Int. J. Surg. 27, 165–175.

NICE, 2008, 2017. Irritable bowel syndrome in adults: diagnosis and management https://www.nice.org.uk/guidance/cg61/chapter/introduction.

NICE, 2012, 2016. Crohn's disease management. https://www.nice.org.uk/guidance/cg152/ifp/chapter/Crohns-disease.

NICE, 2013. Ulcerative colitis management. https://www.nice.org.uk/guidance/CG166/chapter/1-Recommendations#pregnant-women.

NICE, 2015. Coeliac disease: recognition, assessment and management. https://www.nice.org.uk/guidance/ng20/chapter/Context.

NMC, 2015. Standards of competence for registered midwives. https://www.nmc.org.uk/globalassets/sitedocuments/standards/nmc-standards-for-competence-for-registered-midwives.pdf.

Rankin, J., 2017. Physiology in Childbearing: With Anatomy and Related Biosciences, 4th ed. Eslevier, Edinburgh.

Robson, S.E., Waugh, J., 2013. Medical Disorders in Pregnancy: A Manual for Midwives. Wiley-Blackwell, Chichester.

Royal College of Obstetricians and Gynaecologists, 2011. Obstetric Cholestasis Green top guideline no 43. https://www.rcog.org.uk/en/guidelines-research-services/guidelines/gtg43/.

Skubic, J.J., Salim, A., 2017. Emergency general surgery in pregnancy. Trauma Surgery Acute Care Open 2 (1), e000125. http://doi.org/10.1136/tsaco-2017-000125.

Wang, D.Q.H., Portincasa, P.A.M., 2017. Gallstones: Recent Advances in Epidemiology, Pathogenesis, Diagnosis and Management. Nova Biomedical, New York.

CHAPTER 7

Cardiac conditions

Rachel Jokhi and Roobin Jokhi

TRIGGER SCENARIO

Jane is 24 years old and was born with tetralogy of Fallot, which was diagnosed at 2 days of age. She had surgery in a cardiac centre to correct this at 6 months of age, followed by further surgery at age 5 to widen the origin of one of the pulmonary arteries. Jane had regular follow-up with the paediatric cardiology team, who decided to start her on long-term beta blockers for an abnormal heart rhythm. Jane is in a stable relationship and wishes to explore her options about pregnancy but is anxious due to her previous health problems.

Introduction

Pregnancy is a normal physiological event and one that demands rapid and profound physiological adjustments in order to support the growing fetus and prepare the mother for birth. These physiological changes, whilst tolerated well by most women, can prove life threatening for women who are affected by a cardiac condition (Carlin & Alfirevic 2008). This chapter provides a review of the physiology of the changes to the cardiovascular system in pregnancy and identifies the potential risk for women and their babies. The main cardiac conditions, acquired and congenital, will be explored and risk factors for these identified. It will also examine multi-disciplinary management of the condition and consider the midwife's role in the wider multi-disciplinary team in order to provide a holistic and woman-centred approach.

Prevalence of cardiac disease in pregnancy

Cardiac disease complicates approximately 0.2% to 4% of all pregnancies in the western world (Nanda et al 2012), and whilst not common, remains a significant cause of maternal mortality. The 2017 maternal mortality report stated that cardiac disease remained the leading cause of indirect maternal deaths during or up to 6 weeks after the end of pregnancy, with a rate of 2.34 per 100,000 maternities. (Knight et al 2017). Indeed, there has been no significant decrease in the maternal mortality rate from cardiac disease in the last 10 years. Of all the women who died, over 68% had a known medical condition before they started their pregnancy journey. Yet 77% of those who died from cardiac disease were not known to have any pre-existing cardiac problems (Brennand et al 2017). There is therefore a need for all health professionals to be vigilant to the possibility of new-onset or overt cardiac disease in women of childbearing age (Knight et al 2016).

Physiological in pregnancy

The physiological changes to the cardiovascular system during pregnancy take place to facilitate the increased demand for oxygen and nutrients by the utero-placental unit and that of the growing fetus. In normal pregnancy, dramatic changes in cardiovascular physiology occur, initiated by a fall in systemic vascular resistance to 30% to 70% of its pre-conception value by 8 weeks of gestation (Gelson et al 2008). Hormonal changes during pregnancy cause an increase in blood volume starting as early as the fifth week. In the healthy woman, the increase in cardiac output is secondary to a greater stroke volume and higher heart rate. Cardiac output can increase by 30% to 50% by the end of the second trimester of pregnancy. Blood flow to the uterus increases from 50 ml/minute at 10 weeks' gestation to 850 ml/minute at term (Carlin & Alfirevic 2008).

There is a drop in systemic and pulmonary vascular resistance due to prostaglandin production, thus preventing a rise in pulmonary artery pressure from the increased circulating volume. This is beneficial, as a rise in pulmonary artery pressure can be associated with the development of pulmonary oedema and in women with pre-existing cardiac conditions, increase the risk of cardiac failure. The systolic and diastolic pressures fall, reaching their lowest values during the second trimester, before increasing as term approaches, although never reaching pre-pregnancy value (Carlin & Alfirevic 2008).

Physiological changes during labour and following birth

During labour, cardiac output increases by a further 25% to 50% with up to 500 ml of blood returned from the intervillous spaces during contractions (Nelson-Piercy 2002). Cardiac output increases further due to increased heart rate from pain and anxiety and uterine contractions returning blood to the venous system. Blood pressure and oxygen requirements also rise during contractions.

Further increases occur after birth due to a relative hypervolemic state immediately following birth, due to the relief of aortocaval compression from the gravid uterus and auto-transfusion of 300 to 500 ml of blood from the contracted uterus back into the mother's circulation (Nelson-Piercy 2002). Cardiac output, stroke volume and heart rate remain high for 24 hours following birth.

Therefore, the latter stages of labour and the early postpartum period are periods of high risk of cardiac failure (Gelson et al 2008).

> ### Activity
>
> Define the terms *systemic vascular resistance*, *cardiac output* and *stroke volume*.
>
> How do the changes in systemic and pulmonary resistance help balance the increase in cardiac output?
>
> Why are women with a known cardiac disease at higher risk during pregnancy?

Pathophysiology of cardiac disease

Cardiac disease can be classified as either congenital or acquired. In women of childbearing age, acquired disorders are rare; however, the incidence of acquired heart disease is increasing due to older age at first pregnancy and a higher prevalence of cardiovascular risk factors such as hypertension, diabetes, smoking, alcohol intake and obesity. Acquired causes of cardiac disease include rheumatic heart disease, ischaemic heart disease and dissection of the aorta. In addition, increasing global mobility may have an impact on the numbers of childbearing women who may have underlying cardiac disease and who now live in the United Kingdom. This is a contributing factor to the differences in maternal morbidity between ethnic groups (Knight et al 2016).

The commonest congenital heart diseases (CHDs) include ventricular and atrial septal defects and patent ductus arteriosus (PDA). These are mostly diagnosed before pregnancy and are often corrected (Jarvis & Nelson-Piercy 2016). Roberts and Ketchell (2012) suggest that CHD is the leading category of heart disease that midwives will encounter in pregnancy, mainly as a result of improved diagnosis in childhood or early pregnancy and medical advances in the treatments and repair of congenital heart abnormalities, which have led to a significant increase in the number of women with CHD reaching childbearing age. The need to identify women at risk of heart disease and to plan their careful management is an essential aspect of midwifery care.

Acquired cardiac disorders
Rheumatic heart disease

Acquired cardiac disorders occur as a result of a complication of another disease process. The most common cause for childbearing women is as a result of a complication of rheumatic fever as a child resulting from group A streptococcus infection. This may present initially as a respiratory infection or scarlet fever. Morbidity associated with this varies from a mild condition that goes almost unnoticed to an acute illness with a mortality rate of 2% to 3%. Rheumatic heart disease occurs when there has been acute endocardial inflammation and scarring as a result of the infection, resulting in cardiac valve damage (either aortic or mitral). Rheumatic valvular disease comprises 56% to 89% of all cardiovascular disease in pregnancy in developing countries but is relatively rare in the UK (Nanda et al 2012).

Mitral stenosis (MS) is the most common rheumatic valvular disease and is increasingly recognized in migrant women, who may or may not have had the diagnosis made before pregnancy. Damage to the valves means narrowing of the opening and prevention of the valves closing properly. This incomplete closure of the valves results in backflow of the circulating blood in the heart, with impaired circulation and potential for long-term structural damage to the heart. During pregnancy, increases in heart rate, carbon monoxide, red blood cell mass and plasma volume can lead to increased left atrial pressures and cardiac decompensation. Some women with rheumatic MS will present with symptoms for the first time during pregnancy due to these hemodynamic changes. If left untreated, this can lead to further complications such as cardiac hypertrophy and pulmonary oedema and hypertension. Women with valvular heart disease who may have been asymptomatic pre-pregnancy may develop symptoms for the first time in pregnancy due to their increased cardiac output. Stenotic valves are a significant risk factor in pregnancy, as they represent an obstruction to the increased blood flow required in pregnancy. This can lead to ventricular failure, arrhythmias or hypoperfusion (Nelson-Piercy 2015).

Pericarditis is another disease that results in inflammation of the pericardium as a consequence of infection, cardiac injury or an immune response, with reduced perfusion to the heart tissues and resultant scarring. This can mean the heart does not expand sufficiently or stretch due to the scarring, resulting in pain on breathing and generalized chest pain.

Ischaemic heart disease

Ischaemic heart disease is due to inadequate myocardial blood flow as a result of narrowing of the coronary arteries. With complications associated with diet and obesity in industrialized countries, it is becoming increasingly common to meet women who have early signs of ischaemic heart disease as a result of atherosclerosis. Ischaemic heart disease can also be categorized within an umbrella term of *acute coronary syndrome*, which covers different presentations of acute myocardial ischaemia from unstable angina (pain) to myocardial infarction. Myocardial infarction is more commonly known as a *heart attack*, and although rare in pregnancy, maternal mortality may be up to 40% (Wylie & Bryce 2008).

Activity

What is meant by the term *atherosclerosis*?

How does this have an impact on the cardiovascular system?

What complications can result from someone suffering with atherosclerosis?

Individuals with atherosclerosis typically have risk factors, and pregnant women are no exception, with lifestyle factors such as smoking, older maternal age and obesity being particularly important (Burchill et al 2015). The incidence of acute coronary syndrome in pregnancy is an area of debate, but the UK Obstetric Surveillance System (UKOSS) study reported an incidence of 1.7 per 100,000 (Bush et al 2013). Lifestyle issues appear to play an important part in maternal risk from ischaemic heart disease, with all the women who died from ischaemic heart disease having at least one identifiable risk factor. In the 2016 MBRRACE maternal mortality report (Knight et al 2016), smoking was the most common risk factor identified amongst women who died, consistent with other reports of myocardial infarction in pregnancy (Elkayam et al 2012). Age was also an important risk factor. In the UKOSS study, for every year increase in maternal age there was a 20% increase in the risk of myocardial infarction (Bush et al 2013). Pregnancy itself raises the risk of acute myocardial infarction by threefold to fourfold, with the risk being 30 times higher for women over the age of 40

Box 7.1 **Risk factors for ischaemic heart disease**

- Older age
- Smoking
- Obesity
- Diabetes
- Hypertension
- Family history of premature coronary disease
- Hypercholesterolaemia

years compared with women aged less than 20 years (Royal College of Obstetricians and Gynaecologists (RCOG) 2011). The risk factors for ischaemic heart disease are outlined in Box 7.1.

Being overweight or obese was also an important risk factor identified, and the relationship between ischaemic heart disease and obesity with a gradient of increasing risk and weight is extensively documented outside of pregnancy. It is also important to consider that women may have multiple risk factors for ischaemic heart disease, and this clustering of risk factors is also important when assessing risk.

Signs and symptoms of ischaemic heart disease

Knight et al (2016) suggest there remains a reluctance for doctors to diagnose cardiac ischaemia in pregnant women. Clinical presentation in many pregnant or postpartum women is the same as for the general population, with chest discomfort which may radiate to the throat, arms, back and shoulders. The pain may be associated with nausea, sweating and breathlessness or even fainting. However, women in general tend to present with less typical symptoms than men, and the diagnosis can be overlooked. Angina in women is more likely to radiate to the throat, into the back and between the shoulder blades (Canto et al 2007). Women are more likely to report symptoms of feeling hot, breathlessness or experiencing a cold sweat. Some women have these symptoms but no chest pain (Khan et al 2013). Women and health professionals should be aware of cardiac symptoms and their importance.

Activity

What clinical signs and symptoms would be suggestive of ischaemic heart disease?

Why do you think it is challenging to diagnose ischaemic heart disease in pregnant women?

What other conditions might be more commonly thought of as an explanation when considering these symptoms?

Peripartum cardiomyopathy

Cardiomyopathy is a disease of the heart muscle (the myocardium) which affects its size, shape and structure. Peripartum cardiomyopathy (PPCM) is defined as the development of a cardiomyopathy that presents with heart failure secondary to left ventricular failure towards the end of pregnancy or in the immediate postpartum period, in the absence of any other cause of heart failure (Stamatelatou et al 2015). The cause of PPCM is unknown in most cases (RCOG 2011). This is a rare condition but one that carries a high mortality rate of between 25% and 50%. In the 2016 maternal mortality report (Knight et al 2016), nine women, all white, died of PPCM, having developed progressive heart failure in the last month of pregnancy or after birth. The time of their deaths ranged from the day of delivery to 330 days postpartum (median 36 days) (Knight et al 2016), with Silwa et al (2010) suggesting 45% of cases present in the first week postpartum. Whilst rare, Sliwa and Bohm (2014) suggest the incidence of PPCM may be increasing due to factors such as increasing maternal age, increasing numbers of multiple pregnancies associated with reproductive technologies and better recognition and diagnosis. Twenty-five per cent of affected women will be hypertensive.

PPCM is more commonly found in multiparous women and in women with multiple pregnancies. Women may present with heart failure, respiratory failure or even stroke. Initial signs and symptoms may be subtle, but if women continue to present with progressive and persistent breathlessness, palpitations, reduced exercise tolerance, shortness of breath when lying flat and a dry cough (Silwa & Bohm 2014), this should prompt the health professional to investigate further.

Activity

What minor symptoms can a healthy pregnant woman experience as she progresses through pregnancy?

Considering the symptoms described earlier, what other diagnosis may be offered as an explanation to women?

Congenital heart disease

CHDs affect 0.4% to 1.5% of the general population (Greutman & Pieper 2015) and are the most common birth defects. Major advances in open heart surgery have led to rapidly evolving cohorts of adult survivors, and the majority of affected women now survive to childbearing age. The risk of cardiovascular complications during pregnancy and the peripartum period depends on the type of the underlying defect and any co-morbidities. It is important to recognize that these patients are not cured, even if they have had corrective surgery, and many are at high risk of cardiovascular complications and increased risk of premature death Swan (2014).

Risks

One in 125 people is born with CHD (Mandalenakis et al 2017). For women with the condition, pregnancy-induced cardiovascular stress can cause complications such as arrhythmia, heart failure and thromboembolism. The UK Confidential Enquiry (Knight et al 2016) into maternal deaths found that of 910 maternal deaths between 2009 and 2014, 205 (22.5%) were caused by heart disease and a minority from CHD. The European Registry on Heart Disease is the largest published cohort of women with pregnancy complicated by heart disease. In 2012, of 1321 pregnant women with heart disease, 66% had CHD. The overall risk of maternal death in women with CHD is approximately 1%, which is 100 times higher than the background risk for maternal mortality in the developed world (Greutmann & Silversides 2013). Box 7.2 details some of the cardiac and obstetric risks for women with CHD.

The risk of CHD in the children of these women is higher than background, with 3% to 5% having the condition (Bush et al 2013). A UK single-centre study (331 women) showed that preterm labour and pre-labour rupture of membranes were more common (12% and 14%, respectively) than in those without CHD, while the incidence of babies being small for gestational age (less than tenth centile) was 25%, and the neonatal mortality rate was 4% (Gelson et al 2011).

Box 7.2 **Risks for women with congenital heart disease in pregnancy**

Maternal cardiac risk
- Common complications of congenital heart disease
- Arrhythmias
- Heart failure
- Thromboembolic events
- These complications can lead to need for major surgery, disability and premature death

Maternal obstetric risk
Higher incidence of:
- Miscarriage
- Preterm pre-labour rupture of membranes
- Postpartum haemorrhage

From (Cauldwell 2018)

The more common CHDs that may be seen in pregnancy include:

+ Atrial or ventricular septal defects
+ PDA
+ Pulmonary or aortic stenosis (± tetralogy of Fallot)
+ Marfan's syndrome

Atrial or ventricular septal defects

Such defects are characterized by an abnormal opening between the left and right atrium or left and right ventricle. The most common congenital heart lesions in adults are the atrial septal defects, accounting for 10% to 17% of all lesions. Atrial septal defects therefore may present or be detected for the first time in pregnancy. Atrial septal defects are usually not corrected unless the opening is very large, leading to blood moving from the left side of the heart to the right. Over time, there will be subsequent right ventricular overload and dilatation and eventual heart failure. Hypertension and coronary heart disease can make the problem worse (Wylie & Bryce 2008). Ventricular septal defect is one of the most common CHDs. A ventricular septal defect is often detected on routine examination, as it is invariably associated with a loud systolic murmur. For this reason, most significant defects are diagnosed and surgically treated in childhood. Approximately 60% of these will close spontaneously, whilst the remaining 40% will require open heart surgery, usually in infancy (McLean et al 2013).

Patent ductus arteriosus

This is the persistence of the normal fetal structure between the left pulmonary artery and the descending aorta. In utero, blood is oxygenated by the placenta, and therefore the fetal lungs are not required to oxygenate the blood. Normally, in response to increased oxygen tension, as soon as the newborn starts to breathe, the unique contractile elements within its walls cause the ductus arteriosus to functionally close 12 to 24 hours after birth, and it is completely sealed after few months, becoming the ligamentum arteriosum, which remains in the normal adult heart. Persistence of this fetal structure after 10 days of life is considered abnormal. A PDA therefore allows oxygenated blood to flow down a pressure gradient from the aorta to the pulmonary arteries, resulting in some oxygenated blood being diverted away from the tissues in the general circulation. The woman will become short of breath, tire easily on exertion and eventually become cyanotic. If PDA is left untreated, the mortality rate is about 20% by age 20 years, 40% by 40 years and 60% by 60 years as a result of heart failure complicated by pulmonary hypertension (PH) (Sliwa & Bohm 2014).

Pulmonary or aortic stenosis

Pulmonary stenosis is a condition characterized by obstruction to blood flow from the right ventricle to the pulmonary artery. This obstruction is caused by narrowing at one or more points from the right ventricle to the pulmonary artery. Areas of potential narrowing include thickened muscle below the pulmonary valve and stenosis of the valve itself or of the artery just above the valve. The most common form of pulmonary stenosis is obstruction at the valve itself. The right ventricle must therefore work harder to eject blood into the pulmonary artery, which results in a thickening of the muscle of the right ventricle. More severe cases are diagnosed before birth, but some cases are only diagnosed in the newborn period or infancy when it is noticed that the child is cyanosed. In an older child, severe pulmonary valve stenosis can cause shortness of breath at rest or on minimal exertion but is rarely associated with right ventricular failure or sudden death.

Treatment

Children with mild pulmonary valve stenosis rarely require treatment. However, mild pulmonary stenosis in a young infant may progress to more severe degrees and requires careful follow-up. Children with moderate-to-severe degrees of pulmonary stenosis require treatment, the timing of which is often elective and can be performed using a balloon to dilate the narrowed part of the artery. Open heart surgical procedures are required for more complex valves, where balloon dilation is not sufficient therapy.

Some adults with pulmonary stenosis will have had a balloon dilation or surgical opening of the valve. Most of these patients will have had an excellent result and may not need much care or attention as adults. A significant number of these patients will have a significant leak of the pulmonary valve. This can lead to excessive enlargement of the right heart and may eventually need pulmonary valve replacement.

A third group of adults have a moderate amount of pulmonary stenosis and are well. A certain proportion of these people will develop problems, and expert surveillance is recommended. Finally, pulmonary stenosis can present as part of a more complex set of congenital heart anomalies. All such patients require lifelong, expert surveillance and management.

Tetralogy of Fallot

Tetralogy of Fallot is one of the most commonly repaired congenital defects seen in adulthood and represents approximately 5% to 7% of CHDs. It is an abnormality of the heart that has four aspects to it:

1. A large ventricular septal defect
2. Pulmonary stenosis
3. An overriding aorta
4. Right ventricular hypertrophy

In a patient with tetralogy of Fallot, blood can travel across the ventral septal defect from the right ventricle to the left ventricle and out into the aorta. Obstruction in the pulmonary valve leading from the right ventricle to the lung artery prevents the normal amount of blood from being pumped to the lungs. Sometimes the pulmonary valve is completely obstructed and will need to be removed and replaced by a mechanical valve. Consequently, cyanosis is amongst the diagnostic features of this condition in infancy, and open heart surgery is usually performed in infancy to correct this. Lifelong cardiac follow-up is required for individuals who have this condition, because despite surgical advances, the replaced valves may become leaky as the heart grows, leading to pulmonary regurgitation and arrhythmias, causing dizziness and fainting.

Activity

Read the Knight et al (2016) MBRRACE-UK – Saving Lives, Improving Mothers' Care report – Chapter 3, pp. 62–67 at https://www.npeu.ox.ac.uk/downloads/files/mbrrace-uk/reports/MBRRACE-UK%20Maternal%20Report%202016%20-%20website.pdf.

What additional measures are recommended for individuals who have had valve replacement surgery?

Pulmonary hypertension

PH is a progressive elevation of pulmonary artery pressure which, if uncorrected, can lead to right ventricular failure and death. In individuals who are not affected by PH, pulmonary vascular resistance usually decreases in pregnancy (as a result of increasing circulating levels of progesterone) in order to accommodate the increase in maternal circulation and associated increase in cardiac output. In individuals affected by PH, however, this decrease in pulmonary vascular resistance does not occur, and instead the pulmonary circulation is unable to accommodate the increased cardiac output, resulting in increased pulmonary artery pressures, impeded blood flow to the lungs and right ventricle failure.

Diagnosis of PH

PH is usually diagnosed by a combination of history and physical examination in conjunction with non-invasive and invasive investigations. It is classified as pulmonary arterial hypertension, which can be idiopathic, familial, drug/toxin-related or related to connective tissue disorders or to CHD – mainly septal defects – or PH due to left heart disease, lung disease, thromboembolic disease or an unclear aetiology (Elykayam et al 2016).

Prognosis for women with PH

Regardless of the cause, pulmonary arterial hypertension in pregnancy carries an extremely poor prognosis. It is known to be associated with a significantly high mortality rate, between 30% and 56% (Bédard et al 2009; Kiely et al 2010), although there is evidence that it may be as low as 16% in women treated with targeted anti-PH therapies (Pieper et al 2014). There is also an associated miscarriage rate of 40% (Naquib et al 2010).

Acute conditions associated with pregnancy may be complicated by severe PH, such as pulmonary and amniotic fluid embolism. The UK Confidential Enquiry (Knight et al 2016) into maternal deaths found that six women died from pulmonary arterial hypertension, and of these, it was secondary to CHD in two. Labour and the early postpartum period are the most dangerous times for these women due to the changes associated with increased cardiac output and post-partum fluid shift, which may lead to sudden right heart failure and death. Increased mortality rates are not only observed before pregnancy but also in the first months after birth. Indeed Smith et al (2012) suggest the majority of maternal deaths occur during labour or within 1 month postpartum. Emmanuel and Thorne (2015) suggest the risk of mortality remains increased for 6 weeks after the birth.

Care of women with PH

Women with pulmonary arterial hypertension should be counselled about the very high risk of pregnancy and given clear contraceptive advice, as well as advice about interruption of any unintended pregnancy (Hemnes et al 2015). When a woman chooses to continue the pregnancy, she should be immediately referred to a specialized PH centre for management by a multi-disciplinary team that includes a cardiologist experienced in the management of cardiac problems in pregnancy. Each woman will require individual assessment and management according to local specialist experience. Caesarean section as the mode of birth is recommended at around 35 weeks, with monitoring in intensive care for 2 weeks following the birth (Emmanuel & Thorne 2015; Kiely et al 2006; Naquib et al 2010).

Signs and symptoms of cardiac disease

It can be difficult to diagnose early signs and symptoms of cardiac disease in pregnancy, as pregnancy itself produces a similar systemic response. Such signs and symptoms are listed in Box 7.3.

Cardiac disease is usually classified according to the limitations in activity it causes. The New York Heart Association classification of cardiac disease (Table 7.1) is widely used, together with other levels of diagnosis for management planning and prognosis.

Risks to the fetus

The risks to the fetus can be considerable depending upon the cardiac condition that affects the mother. These include a higher incidence of fetal growth restriction, preterm birth, intracranial haemorrhage, fetal and neonatal death and a risk of CHD in infants, with a risk of 3% to 50% (against a background risk of 0.8% in others who do not have

---

Box 7.3 Sign and symptoms of cardiac disease

- Overwhelming fatigue – due to the heart being unable to transport oxygenated blood efficiently to meet the metabolic requirements of the tissues
- Shortness of breath – severe enough to limit normal activity
- Palpitations – due to heart arrhythmias
- A bounding, collapsing pulse – due to associated tachycardia without the corresponding increase in cardiac output
- Chest pain associated with activity – due to ischaemic heart disease
- Peripheral oedema – due to inadequate venous return

Table 7.1: New York classification of cardiovascular disease

Class	Classification
I	No limitation of physical activity. No shortness of breath, fatigue, or heart palpitations with ordinary physical activity.
II	Slight limitation of physical activity. Shortness of breath, fatigue, or heart palpitations with ordinary physical activity, but patients are comfortable at rest.
III	Marked limitation of activity. Shortness of breath, fatigue, or heart palpitations with less than ordinary physical activity, but patients are comfortable at rest.
IV	Severe to complete limitation of activity. Shortness of breath, fatigue, heart palpitations with any physical exertion and symptoms appear even at rest.

congenital cardiac disease) (Cauldwell et al 2018). Pre-conceptual counselling can offer women and their partners the opportunity to discuss any concerns and risks regarding their pregnancy and the effect this can have on them and their unborn baby.

Pre-conceptual counselling

The UK Confidential Enquiry into Maternal Deaths (Knight et al 2016) highlighted the importance of pre-conception counselling, and the European Society of Cardiology guidance (2018) emphasizes that counselling before conception should be readily available at the transition from paediatric to adult cardiac care, ideally by referral to a combined cardiology-obstetric clinic. Informed maternal decision-making is crucial, and there is a clear need for individualized care, taking into account not only the medical condition but also the emotional and cultural context, psychological issues and ethical challenges, including whether or not to continue with a pregnancy. However, women with cardiac disease can expect a successful pregnancy outcome. Specialized multi-disciplinary pre-conception counselling should be available to all women of reproductive age with congenital or acquired heart disease in order to empower them in making choices (RCOG 2011).

All women of childbearing age referred for a valve operation before pregnancy should receive pre-pregnancy counselling by a team (cardiologist, obstetrician, midwife and relevant others, including anaesthetist) with expertise in managing patients with valvular heart disease during pregnancy (RCOG 2008; Regitz-Zagrosek et al 2018).

Issues considered before pregnancy include review of medication and commencement of folic acid, dietary advice, smoking cessation and a dental visit to minimize the risk of infection and invasive dental treatment during pregnancy. Other lifestyle issues include avoidance of tobacco, drugs and alcohol.

Activity

What are the aims of pre-pregnancy care?

Why is pre-pregnancy counselling important for women with known cardiac disease?

Read Faculty of Sexual and Reproductive Healthcare Clinical Effectiveness Unit (2014). *Contraceptive Choices for Women with Cardiac Disease* at *https://www.fsrh.org/standards-and-guidance/documents/ceu-guidance-contraceptive-choices-for-women-with-cardiac/*. Ideally, when should contraceptive advice be discussed to prevent pregnancy in women with CHD?

Antenatal care

Occasionally, women without a history of heart disease might present for the first time in pregnancy with a major cardiac event; therefore careful midwifery assessment can aid in the diagnosis. This begins at the first midwifery appointment when a woman's booking history or physical assessment may reveal risk factors. Where these or deviations from normal are identified, midwives have a responsibility to refer women to the most appropriate health professional (Nursing and Midwifery Council 2013) and to ensure that women understand the reasons for referral to a consultant obstetrician.

Investigations

Women who present with cardiac symptoms in pregnancy are referred to a cardiologist for full cardiac investigations as follows: an electrocardiogram, an echocardiogram and a series of laboratory tests including cardiac enzymes and electrolytes. Although the physiological burden of normal pregnancy can cause breathlessness and palpitations, any new onset requires careful evaluation, often with referral to the cardiac and/or obstetric team.

Multi-disciplinary care and surveillance

All women should be seen by a multi-disciplinary team which includes the midwife, the obstetrician, a cardiologist and an anaesthetist, ideally in a joint clinic to minimize the number of visits required and to facilitate integrated care records, which can help keep track of appointments and facilitate communication between different healthcare providers At each antenatal visit clinical assessment should include measurement of blood pressure and pulse, heart rhythm, auscultation of heart sounds and lung bases to exclude any pulmonary oedema, maternal oxygen saturations, proteinuria and fetal growth. It is also important to discuss diet, particularly if women are on diuretics and require low-sodium and high-potassium diets in order to prevent electrolyte imbalance. Prevention of anaemia is also vital, as reduction in oxygen-carrying capacity of the red blood cells will further exacerbate the stress that the heart is under. Controlling weight gain is particularly important to prevent further cardiac stress, and the midwife may need to consider referral to a dietician.

Assessment of fetal wellbeing is paramount, and the European Society of Cardiology (2018) and the RCOG (2011) recommend fetal growth monitoring using ultrasound and Doppler, particularly if a woman is taking beta blockers, as maternal heart disease is associated with an increased risk of fetal growth restriction. Ultrasound screening of the fetus at 11 to 14 weeks' gestation may be advised to detect abnormal nuchal translucency, which has a strong association with CHD in the fetus (Cauldwell et al 2018).

The antenatal period is also a time for review of medications, as some drugs, for example, warfarin, are teratogenic and therefore cannot be used in the first trimester of pregnancy due to the risk of skeletal defects, intracranial haemorrhage and abnormalities of the central nervous system.

Activity

Review your local guidelines for the treatment of pregnant women with cardiac conditions. Which drugs are commonly used to treat cardiac conditions?

Are there any adverse effects or contraindications from taking these drugs in pregnancy, and can they be taken whilst breastfeeding?

Research the fetal risks of newer anticoagulant drugs.

Labour

Most women with CHD can expect and are typically offered as normal a birth as possible, including spontaneous onset of labour. However, in general women are advised to have their birth in hospital and to attend as soon as in labour.

Women with cardiac disease often have quick and uncomplicated labours, but it is essential that physiological and psychological stress is kept to a minimum. Reviewing and discussing pain relief in the antenatal period can be helpful when planning care in labour, as many women may be encouraged to have an epidural, as this decreases cardiac output and causes vasodilation, therefore reducing venous resistance and reducing cardiac stress. Similarly, women may be encouraged to give birth in an upright or left lateral position to reduce the impact of aortocaval compression (Wylie & Bryce 2008). Close monitoring is required throughout and should include maternal pulse and heart rate plus pulse oximetry and fluid balance. Oxygen therapy may also be required, depending on the severity of the cardiac condition and its effects on the woman.

Personalized care

Despite the highly complex conditions the midwife should still continue to facilitate as normal a birthing process as possible, depending on how well the woman is. As the mother with cardiac disease may experience considerable psychological stress, anxiety and fear, the midwife has a crucial role in providing individualized woman-centred care, which includes giving a balanced account of the progression of labour and likely outcome and providing emotional support for the woman and her partner. Involving the woman and her partner in decisions and preferences about their care can help provide the woman with a sense of control that she could potentially feel she has lost as a result of having a serious medical condition. It is the midwife's professional duty of care to act as an advocate for the woman at all times (Nursing and Midwifery Council (NMC) 2018) and provide woman-centred care to all women, irrespective of risk status (Magill-Cuerden 2005).

Both Regitz-Zagrosek et al (2018) and RCOG (2011) recommend active management of the third stage as women with cardiac disease are at greater risk of having a postpartum haemorrhage then if they did not have a cardiac condition. However, ergometrine is contraindicated because it can cause significant and immediate vasoconstriction and a systemic rapid rise in blood pressure. Oxytocin is therefore the drug of choice, although this can cause hypotension and tachycardia and so is recommended to be given as a slow intravenous infusion, rather than an intramuscular injection (Regitz-Zagrosek et al 2018).

Postnatal period

The immediate postnatal period is a high-risk period, as many haemodynamic changes occur concurrently. Intensity of maternal monitoring depends upon the underlying congenital lesion, predisposition to arrhythmia and the presence of symptoms of heart failure. The midwife should remain vigilant in monitoring the mother for any signs of infection that would increase her risk of an adverse outcome. Medications are reviewed and adjusted at this time, and follow-up review can be discussed with the woman.

Breastfeeding

Midwives should strive to support informed choice. Most drugs used in the treatment of cardiac disease enter the breast milk, but women can be reassured that breastfeeding is safe with most cardiac medications. The midwife should be familiar with these drugs and their compatibility with breastfeeding in order to support women in their choice of infant feeding.

Look back on the trigger scenario.

> *Jane is 24 years old and was born with tetralogy of Fallot diagnosed at 2 days of age. She had surgery in a cardiac centre to correct this at 6 months of age, followed by further surgery at age 5 to widen the origin of one of the pulmonary arteries. She had regular follow-up with the paediatric cardiology team, who put her on beta blockers for an abnormal heart rhythm. Jane has been in a stable relationship and wishes to explore her options about pregnancy but is anxious about this due to her previous problems.*

Now that you are familiar with the issues in relation to cardiac disease in pregnancy, you should have insight into how the scenario relates to the evidence. The jigsaw model will now be used to explore the trigger scenario in more depth.

Effective communication

Effective identification, investigation, management and support for women with cardiac disease in pregnancy are frequently fraught with difficulties. Therefore, it can be challenging for midwives to be sure that women have a sufficient understanding about their condition to make valid choices. Questions that arise from this scenario might include: Does Jane wish to undertake a potentially risky pregnancy? If she does decide to proceed, can she make informed decisions about her care? What questions could the midwife ask Jane to establish her prior understanding about her congenital heart condition? How could Jane's response enhance information-sharing? What methods can the midwife use to ensure that Jane understands any new information?

Woman-centred care

In women who have had corrected congenital cardiac disease, cardiac function in pregnancy can be variable. Similarly, women's responses to being informed about potential complications to the pregnancy, which encompass both issues related to their own health and that of their baby, will be determined by a range of factors such as their cultural beliefs and their perceptions of their medical condition. Questions that may be asked in relation to this scenario are: How might continuity of care from a known midwife benefit Jane in addition to reviews with a consultant obstetrician? What support networks does Jane have, and how can these help Jane feel that she will be well cared for during and after her pregnancy? How can the midwife ensure that she is meeting Jane's physical, emotional and social needs?

Using best evidence

In response to the consistent numbers of women identified in recent confidential enquiries who have died as a result of cardiac disease, the Royal College of Obstetricians and Gynaecologists published Good Practice Guide No.13 – Cardiac Disease in Pregnancy (RCOG 2011). They acknowledge that there is a lack of evidence-based guidelines to assist in planning the management of affected pregnancies. The purpose of the Good Practice guidance is 'to provide a summary of current expert opinion as an interim measure, with the hope that these opinions will be supplemented by objective evidence in due course' (RCOG 2011:2). Questions that arise from the scenario might include: How can midwives ensure that the information they share with women is the most relevant to women's needs? How much knowledge does Jane already possess about how best to proceed before pregnancy? Can the midwife reassure Jane that her care in pregnancy will be managed by clinicians who are up to date with the relevant issues? Will the paucity of research-based guidelines impact on Jane's ability to take ownership of the management of her pregnancy?

Professional and legal issues

Midwives are responsible for practising in accordance with the Code (NMC 2018), their employer's policies and the law. Providing high-quality care for women with potentially life-threatening conditions such as congenital cardiac disease requires adequate access to information technology, being informed about the progression of the pregnancy and access to the relevant specialist clinicians involved in the care of these women should questions or issues arise during the pregnancy. Questions that arise from the scenario might include: In what ways can detailed, contemporaneous documentation support professional and accountable midwifery care? Have the clinicians involved in Jane's care established parameters regarding her condition that the midwife can logically follow to determine whether Jane's management is stable? What are the midwife's responsibilities if Jane declined investigations or treatments in relation to her pre-existing condition? Who is the point of contact for the midwife from senior management for any concerns that she may have regarding Jane's care?

Team working

It is crucial to provide safe and effective care in any complex medical condition, especially in the scenario described. The basis for this is close liaison between the members of the multi-professional team, regardless of whether they have direct or indirect contact with the woman. Questions that could arise from the scenario include: Which clinical disciplines might be involved in the care of a woman with corrected congenital cardiac disease? How does a specialist clinic with continuity of care provided by midwives and doctors help improve outcomes? If such a clinic is not available, what could the midwife do to ensure Jane's needs are being met? In what circumstances might the midwife need to escalate Jane's care to another health professional?

Clinical dexterity

Midwives are responsible for ensuring that maternal observations such as heart rate, blood pressure measurements and urinalysis are performed accurately and appropriately and any concerns are escalated in a timely manner. The other key role is being able to assess fetal wellbeing in such a high-risk pregnancy. Questions that might arise in relation to Jane's situation include: What parameters should the midwife use to be able to assess Jane's adaptation to pregnancy? Have these been clearly documented and an appropriate plan made as to which clinical factors would trigger a referral to the appropriate clinician? Would any of Jane's medications alter the clinical signs that a midwife would normally use to assess maternal wellbeing? What key clinical considerations need to be combined in the assessment of Jane's obstetric health and emotional state? How could the use of an individualized fetal growth chart help the midwife detect fetal growth restriction or oligohydramnios?

Models of care

Women who have complex medical conditions in pregnancy are likely to experience multi-professional care. A balance still needs to be struck between the input required for their ongoing medical care and the need to adapt their care to allow it to be individualized and personal. Questions that arise from the scenario might include: What is Jane's perception of her care in pregnancy with regard to the role of the midwife? How might continuity of carer benefit women such as Jane, who might have appointments with a number of different health professionals? Is there scope in the midwifery staffing rotas so that Jane could be cared for by a familiar midwife in the hospital setting?

Safe environment

A key role of midwives is to act as advocates for their patients to ensure that women feel they are clinically well looked after, as well as making sure they are emotionally secure. Questions that arise from the scenario might include: Is Jane going to be cared for in the most appropriate environment for her level of needs? Have Jane's opinions and wishes been acknowledged and taken into consideration? How does the midwife contend with a situation where Jane wishes to deviate from a medically recommended care plan for labour or delivery which she feels may not be safe?

Promotes health

For some people with chronic medical conditions, despite being in the health system for many years, they may not be fully aware of how their lifestyle choices influence their overall health and wellbeing. The midwife has an important role to play in educating pregnant women with complex medical needs and sharing information to optimize physical care of the mother and baby. Questions that arise from the scenario might include: How might Jane's lifestyle affect her pre-existing cardiac condition? What impact, if any, would this have on her risks with regard to maternal and perinatal morbidity and mortality? Can any modifiable risk factors be identified that could improve or ameliorate the risks associated with a future pregnancy?

Further scenarios

The following scenarios enable you to consider how specific situations influence the care the midwife provides. Use the jigsaw model to explore the issues raised in the scenario.

SCENARIO 1

Monica is a 39-year-old woman with a high body mass index (BMI) who has a history of hypertension and poorly controlled type 2 diabetes who conceived spontaneously. She was regularly followed up in the combined diabetes antenatal clinic and had an emergency caesarean section for pre-eclampsia at 35 weeks. Two weeks later, she phoned the midwife reporting symptoms of breathlessness and ankle swelling, which she said predated the pregnancy. The midwife urged Monica to attend the general practitioner (GP) surgery, and thereafter she was urgently referred to the cardiologists. Investigations revealed a severe dilated cardiomyopathy for which she received treatment, and her symptoms improved to allow her home. She was followed up in the cardiology clinic after 3 months at which time she was found to have moderate left ventricular function at 30% to 40% of normal.

Women with cardiac risk factors, for example, older maternal age or obesity, should optimize their pre-pregnancy condition to ensure that they are able to minimize both maternal and perinatal morbidity and mortality. Women should have the opportunity to make informed decisions regarding their care and treatment via access to evidence-based information. These choices should be recognized as an integral part of the decision-making process. Verbal information should be supplemented with written information or audio-visual media.

Questions that could be asked are:
1. Did Monica seek any pre-conceptual advice before embarking on a pregnancy?
2. What questions could the midwife ask Monica to establish her level of understanding about how her pre-morbid health conditions would affect the pregnancy?
3. Were the risk factors for a high-risk pregnancy correctly identified, and was Monica referred into the appropriate setting for her pregnancy care?
4. What steps could the midwife take to minimize the risks to Monica's pregnancy?
5. What symptoms and signs could the midwife use to ascertain that Monica's symptoms warranted referral for further assessment?

SCENARIO 2

Deidre is 41 years old and was in her fifth pregnancy, having had four previous normal deliveries, the last being 11 years previously. The pregnancy was uneventful until 34 weeks when she developed chest pain. The pain had been off and on over 3 days and radiated into her back and left arm. Deidre was known to smoke and had declined smoking cessation, has a family history of ischaemic heart disease and has a history of hypertension. When she was assessed in the local emergency department, her risk factors for coronary disease were elicited and her electrocardiogram (ECG) was reviewed and felt to be abnormal, although her troponin levels (a marker for cardiac muscle damage) was normal. She was transferred to a tertiary centre with access to cardiac catheterization services, and the obstetric team was informed. Extensive coronary artery atherosclerosis and a thrombosed left anterior descending artery were found. Over the next 2 days she was stabilized and proceeded to have an emergency caesarean section at 34+4 weeks. Three months after delivery, Deidre underwent triple bypass surgery, and she is currently symptom free.

Practice point

The woman had multiple risk factors for ischaemic heart disease. The history elicited by the emergency department was suggestive of cardiac pain, and the appropriate referral was made. When assessing a woman with chest pain, care should be given to review the presenting symptoms the woman had before she was given analgesia, and abnormal ECGs should not be ignored. If the history is consistent with ischaemia, a normal ECG and/or negative troponin test do not exclude the diagnosis, and further investigation should be undertaken. It is of paramount importance that a formal diagnosis is made in a woman presenting with chest pain rather than simply using a negative troponin test to exclude a diagnosis and then discharging the woman.

Questions that could be asked are:

1. What were Deidre's feelings about a pregnancy many years after her last child?
2. How could the midwife educate Deidre about the risks of a pregnancy given her personal history of smoking and her family history of ischaemic heart disease?
3. What clinical signs could the midwife look for at each visit to assess Deidre's physical wellbeing?
4. Did the events leading to the delivery affect Deidre's relationship with the baby in the initial days and weeks postnatally?
5. If she was certain that she did not wish to become pregnant again, had Deidre considered reliable and effective contraception appropriate to her characteristics to prevent future pregnancy?

Conclusion

Pregnancy is a normal physiological event and one that demands rapid and profound physiological adjustments. These physiological changes, whilst tolerated well by most women, can prove life threatening for women who are affected by a cardiac condition. Early involvement of senior clinicians from the obstetric, cardiology and midwifery multi-disciplinary team is important, wherever a pregnant or postpartum woman presents with suspected cardiac disease. Women without a history of heart disease might present with a major cardiac event for the first time at any point in or following pregnancy. Midwives play a key role in identifying the risk factors, signs and symptoms of cardiac disease in order to refer women for specialist care and ensure safe and effective care for mothers and their babies.

Resources

Arrhythmia Alliance www.arrhythmiaalliance.org.uk

British Heart Foundation https://www.bhf.org.uk/

Cardiomyopathy Association www.cardiomyopathy.org

European Society of Cardiology https://www.escardio.org/static_file/Escardio/ Guidelines/publications/PREGN%20Guidelines-Pregnancy-FT.pdf Guidelines on the management of cardiovascular diseases during pregnancy.

LactMed/TOXNET https://toxnet.nlm.nih.gov/newtoxnet/lactmed.htm Free advice from the National Institute of Health on the safety of drug use when breastfeeding

Royal College of Obstetricians and Gynaecologists https://www.rcog.org.uk/ globalassets/documents/guidelines/goodpractice13cardiacdiseaseand-pregnancy.pdf Practice guidance on the management of cardiac disease in pregnancy.

The Somerville Foundation http://www.thesf.org.uk Free information for patients with GUCH (grown up congenital heart), including information about pregnancy.

UK Teratology Information Service http://rdtc.nhs.uk/services/teratology Free advice from the Regional Drug and Therapeutic Centre.

References

Bédard, E., Dimopoulos, K., Gatzoulis, M.A., 2009. Has there been any progress made on pregnancy outcomes among women with pulmonary arterial hypertension? Eur. Heart J. 30 (3), 256–265.

Brennand, J., Northridge, R., Scott, H., Walker, N., (2017) Addressing the Heart of the Issue: Good clinical practice in the shared obstetric and cardiology care of women of childbearing age, Royal College of Physicians and Surgeons, Glasgow. https://rcpsg.ac.uk/media/news/1808/addressing-the-heart-of-the-issue.pdf.

Burchill, L.J., Lameijer, H., Ross-Hesselink, J., et al., 2015. Pregnancy Risks in women with pre-existing coronary artery diseas or following acute coronary syndrome. Heart 101 (7), heart.bmj.com/content/101/7/525.

Bush, N., Nelson-Piercy, C., Spak, P., et al., 2013. Myocardial Infacrtion in pregnancy and the postpartum in the UK. Eur. J. Prev. Cardiol. 20 (1), 12–20.

Canto, J.G., Goldberg, R.J., Hand, M.M., et al., 2007. Symptom presentation of women with acute coronary syndromes: myth vs reality. Arch. Intern. Med. 167 (22), 2405–2413.

Carlin, A., Alfirevic, Z., 2008. Physiological changes of pregnancy and monitoring. Best Pract. Res. Clin. Obstet. Gynaecol. 22 (5), 801–823.

Cauldwell, M., Dos Santos, F., Steer, P., et al., 2018. Pregnancy in women with congenital heart disease. BMJ 360, doi:10.1136/bmj.k478. [Peer Reviewed Journal] British Medical Journal Publishing Group.

Elkayam, U., Jalnapurkar, S., Barakat, M., 2012. Peripartum cardiomyopathy. Cardiol. Clin. 30 (3), 435–440.

Emmanuel, Y., Thorne, S., 2015. Heart disease in pregnancy. Best Pract. Res. Clin. Obstet. Gynaecol. 29 (5), 579–597.

European Society of Cardiology – Management of Cardiovascular Disease During Pregnancy, 2018. https://www.escardio.org/Guidelines/Clinical-Practice-Guidelines/Cardiovascular-Diseases-during-Pregnancy-Management-of.

Faculty of Sexual and Reproductive Healthcare Clinical Effectiveness Unit (2014). Contraceptive Choices for women with cardiac disease. https://www.fsrh.org/documents/ceu-guidance-contraceptive-choices-for-women-withcardiac/ceuguidancecontraceptivechoiceswomencardiacdisease.pdf.

Gelson, E., Curry, R., Gatzoulis, M.A., et al., 2011. Effect of maternal heart disease on fetal growth. Obstet. Gynecol. 117, 886–891. doi:10.1097/AOG.0b013e31820cab69. 21422861.

Gelson, E., Gatzoulis, M., Steer, P.J., et al., 2008. Tetralogy of Fallot: maternal and neonatal outcomes. BJOG 115, 398–402.

Greutmann, M., Pieper, P., 2015. Pregnancy in women with congenital heart disease. Eur. Heart J. 36, 2491–2499. doi:10.1093/eurheartj/ehv288.

Greutmann, M., Silversides, C.K., 2013. The ROPAC registry: a multicentre collaboration on pregnancy outcomes in women with heart disease. Eur. Heart J. 34, 634–635. doi:10.1093/eurheartj/ehs335. 23048193.

Hemnes, A., Kiely, D., et al., 2015. Statement on pregnancy in pulmonary hypertension from the Pulmonary Vascular Research Institute. Pulm. Circ. 5 (3), 435–465.

Jarvis, S., Nelson-Piercy, C., 2010. Cardiac Diseases complicating pregnancy in Anaesthesia and Intensive Care Medicine. 11 (8), pp. 305–309.

Khan, N.A., Daskalopoulou, S.S., Karp, I., et al., 2013. Sex differences in acute coronary syndrome symptom presentation in young patients. JAMA Intern. Med. 173 (20), 1863–1871. doi:10.1001/jamainternmed.2013.10149.

Kiely, D.G., Condliffe, R., et al., 2010. Improved survival in pregnancy and pulmonary hypertension using a multiprofessional approach. BJOG 117 (5), 565–574.

Kiely, D., Elliott, C., Webster, V., Stewart, P., 2006. Pregnancy and Pulmonary Hypertension: new approached to management. In: Steer, P., Gatzoulis, M., Baker, P. (Eds.), Heart Disease in Pregnancy. RCOG Press, London.

Knight, M., Nair, M., Tuffnell, D., et al. on behalf of MBRRACE-UK., Eds. (2016). Saving Lives, Improving Mothers' Care – Surveillance of maternal deaths in the UK 2012-14 and lessons learned to inform maternity care from the UK and Ireland Confidential Enquiries into Maternal Deaths and Morbidity 2009-14. Oxford, National Perinatal Epidemiology Unit, University of Oxford.

Knight, M., Nair, M., Tuffnell, D., et al. on behalf of MBRRACE-UK. (Eds.), 2017. Saving Lives, Improving Mothers' Care – Lessons learned to inform maternity care from the UK and Ireland Confidential Enquiries into Maternal Deaths and Morbidity 2013–15. Oxford: National Perinatal Epidemiology Unit, University of Oxford 2017.

Magill-Cuerden, J., 2005. Making midwifery-led care inclusive care. Br. J. Midwifery 13 (4), 214.

Mandalenakis, Z., Rosengren, A., Skoglund, K., et al., 2017. Survivorship in children and young adults with congenital heart disease in Sweden. JAMA Intern. Med. 177, 224–230. doi:10.1001/jamainternmed.2016.7765. 27992621.

McLean, M., Bu'Lock, F.A., Robson, S.E., 2013. Heart disease. In: Robson, S.E., Waugh, J. (Eds.), Medical Disorders in Pregnancy: A Manual for Midwives. Wiley Blackwell, Chichester, pp. 43–68, (Chapter 4).

Nanda, S., Nelson-Piercy, C., Mackillup, L., 2012. Cardiac disease in pregnancy. Clin. Med. (Northfield Il) 12 (6), 553–560.

Naquib, M.A., Dob, D.P., Gatzoulis, M.A., 2010. A functional understanding of moderate to complex congenital heart disease and the impact of pregnancy. Part II. Int. J. Obstet. Anesth. 19, 306–312.

Nelson-Piercy, C., 2002. Heart disease in pregnancy. Acta Anaesthesiol. Belg. 53 (4), 321–326.

Nelson-Piercy, C., 2015. Handbook of Obstetric Medicine (Vol. Fifth Edition). CRC Press, Boca Raton, FL.

Nursing and Midwifery Council, 2013. Midwives Rules and Standards. NMC, London.

Nursing and Midwifery Council (2018) The Code (amended) NMC London.

Pieper, P., Lameeijer, H., Hoendermis, E., 2014. Pregnancy and Pulmonary Hypertension in Best Practice and Research in Clinical Obstetrics and Gynaecology. 28 (4), pp. 579–591.

Regitz-Zagrosek, V., Roos-Hesselink, J., Bauersachs, J., et al. (2018) 2018 ESC Guidelines for the management of cardiovascular diseases during pregnancy European Society of Cardiology https://www.escardio.org/Guidelines/Clinical-Practice-Guidelines/Cardiovascular-Diseases-during-Pregnancy-Management-of.

Roberts, R., Ketchell, A., 2012. Clinical assessment of women with cardiovascular abnormalities. Br. J. Midwifery 20 (6), 246–251.

Roos-Hesselink, J.W., Ruys, T.P., Stein, J.I., et al., 2013. Outcome of pregnancy in patients with structural or ischaemic heart disease: results of a registry of the European Society of Cardiology. Eur. Heart J. 34, 657–665. doi:10.1093/eurheartj/ehs270. 22968232.

Royal College Obstetricians Gynaecologists (2011) Cardiac Disease and Pregnancy: Good Practice No.13 https://www.rcog.org.uk/globalassets/documents/guidelines/goodpractice13cardiacdiseaseandpregnancy.pdf.

Sliwa, K., Bohm, M., 2014. Incidence and prevalence of pregnancy-related heart disease. Cardiovasc. Res. 101 (4), 554–560.

Smith, J.S., Mueller, J., Daniels, C.J., 2012. Pulmonary arterial hypertension in the setting of pregnancy: a case series and standard treatment approach. Lung 190 (2), 155–160.

Stamatelatou, M., Walker, F., Pandya, B., 2015. A contemporary review of peripartum cardiomyopathy. Br. J. Midwifery 23 (6), 394–400.

Swan, L., 2014. Congenital Heart Disease in pregnancy. Best Pract. Res. Clin. Obstet. Gynaecol. 28 (4), 495–506.

Wylie, L., Bryce, H. (2008) The Midwives' Guide to Key Medical Conditions Churchill Livingstone / Elsevier Edinburgh.

CHAPTER 8

Infections in pregnancy and childbearing

TRIGGER SCENARIO

Sara and Mike are delighted when a pregnancy test confirms that Sara is pregnant with their second baby. Despite feeling excited, Sara is also worried. She gave birth to George at 34 weeks' gestation, and he required treatment on the neonatal unit for an infection. That was a worrying time for the couple, and Sara blamed herself for George's illness. As she makes a note of the first appointment with her midwife, she wonders what she can do to prevent a similar situation occurring this time.

Introduction

Infections during pregnancy, childbearing and the postnatal period can have wide-ranging physical, psychosocial and emotional consequences for women, their babies and families and the people who provide their care. Many types and causes of infection can arise during or shortly after pregnancy; some such as chorioamnionitis are directly related to pregnancy, whereas others such as chest infections may be indirectly related. Some maternal infections increase the risk of perinatal infection. Despite antenatal screening and immunization programmes, confidential enquiries into maternal and perinatal deaths continue to report infection-related mortalities (Draper et al 2018; Knight et al 2017). The National Health Services (NHS) Infectious Diseases in Pregnancy Programme (IDPP) (Public Health England (PHE) 2016) offers screening to all pregnant women to identify and treat some of these conditions (HIV, hepatitis B and syphilis) and as a consequence reduce the risk of mother-to-baby transmission. However, some particularly vulnerable women book late for pregnancy care because of cultural barriers or chaotic or disadvantaged lifestyles (PHE 2013), thus missing opportunities for timely interventions.

This chapter provides a brief outline of the physiology relating to the body's ability to resist infection and an overview of the infectious diseases included in the IDPP. It also includes influenza and group B streptococcal infection since these can have a significant impact on women's experiences of childbearing and current midwifery care. For care of a woman with suspected sepsis, see Volume 6, Chapter 11 in the *Midwifery Essentials* series.

Immunity

The human body normally protects itself against infection through immunity. Intrinsic, non-specific immunity from infection is present from birth and includes factors such as the skin, digestive enzymes and phagocytes with the blood. Immunity may also be acquired through active or passive mechanisms, offering protection against specific organisms. Active immunity develops through a person's own immune system reacting to antigens on an infecting organism that has entered the body as a result of infection or vaccination. This reaction triggers antibody and cell-mediated specific protective responses, which enable the body to react rapidly to subsequent infections. Active immunity is generally long-lasting but is not 100% effective, and some people, for whom vaccination is ineffective or contraindicated, may rely on population (herd) immunity for protection. In contrast, passive immunity, such as the vertical, transplacental transfer of antibodies from mother to fetus or through administering blood products such as immunoglobulins, provides temporary protection (PHE 2013).

Activity

What is population (herd) immunity?
    Find out about vaccination programmes that rely on this strategy.

Viral infections

Viral infections can be a major cause of maternal and fetal or neonatal morbidity and mortality. Infections can be transmitted to the fetus vertically through the placenta, during labour and birth through vaginal secretions and blood, and potentially through direct contact or breast milk in the postnatal period. Hepatitis and HIV are two of these viral infections that have significance for childbearing women and their babies.

Viral hepatitis

Hepatitis is damage or inflammation of the liver that can be harmful for childbearing women, their babies and their carers. There are many causative factors for hepatitis, including infective and non-infective. Viruses that primarily affect the liver (hepatotrophic viruses) include hepatitis A (HAV), B (HBV), C (HCV), D (HDV) and E (HEV). Viral hepatitis is a notifiable disease under the Public Health (Infectious Diseases) Act 1988 (PHE 2017). Symptoms of hepatitis may include fatigue, loss of appetite, nausea, pyrexia, abdominal pain (particularly in the right upper quadrant) and jaundice (Bothamley & Boyle 2015). This section focuses on HBV and HCV, which have the greatest significance for current midwifery practice in the UK.

Hepatitis B

Worldwide, HBV is the most common variety of chronic hepatitis (Silasi et al 2015). It is present in blood and body fluids of an infected person and can remain alive for up to 7 days in dried blood (Bothamley & Boyle 2015). The average incubation period is 60 to 90 days (PHE 2017). It is highly infectious and can cause short-term illness, although some people develop a chronic infection, resulting in cirrhosis of the liver, liver cancer, liver failure and death.

Pregnant women with chronic hepatitis may experience 'flares' and should have regular liver function tests during pregnancy and the postnatal period (Silasi et al 2015). HBV infection during pregnancy can cause severe disease for the mother and chronic infection for the baby (PHE 2017), although it is not associated with congenital malformations or mortality (Silasi et al 2015). Age is associated with likely progression of the infection: 90% of infected babies develop chronic infections compared with around 5% of adults (PHE 2017). Women who are highly infectious have a 70% to 90% risk of passing the infection to their baby during the perinatal period, compared with 10% of infected mothers who are not highly infectious (Department of Health (DH) 2011). Serological markers determine the current status of the infection, with a high viral load (VL) indicating a significant risk for transmission.

Fetal infection is less common, and breastfeeding is not a significant risk factor (Silasi et al 2015). The main aim of management is to minimize the risk of mother-to-baby transmission. Since the risks to the fetus are 'likely to be negligible', vaccination for pregnant or breastfeeding women who pose a definite risk for HBV infection is not contraindicated (PHE 2017:20). Materno-fetal transfer of antibodies can be particularly effective during the third trimester, although there is currently insufficient evidence to support antenatal immunization against HBV to improve newborn outcomes (Eke et al 2017).

Serological markers for HBV

+ Hepatitis B surface antigen (HBsAg) serum levels are high in HBV infections and indicate that the person is infectious. Chronic infection is diagnosed when HBsAg is present for over 6 months (Krajden et al 2005).
+ In response to the infection, the body naturally produces anti-HBsAg antibodies.
+ Hepatitis B surface antibody (anti-HBs) in the blood usually indicates recovery from HBV and immunity. Anti-HBs is also present after successful HBV vaccination (Centers for Disease Control and Prevention (CDC) 2018a).
+ Total hepatitis B core antibody (anti-HBc) is detectable from the time of onset of symptoms and persists for life.
+ Immunoglobulin M (IgM) antibody to hepatitis B core antigen (IgM anti-HBc) indicates acute or recent infection.
+ Hepatitis B e antigen (HBeAg) levels indicate viral replication and high infectivity.
+ Hepatitis B e antibody (HBeAb or anti-HBe) indicates clearance of the HBV in association with anti-viral therapy and lowering levels of HBV (CDC 2018a).

For a summary of the serum markers for HBV, see Table 8.1.

Implications for midwifery practice

The prevalence of HBV in the UK is low, at around 0.4%, although inner-city areas may have rates of 1% or higher (PHE 2017). The risk of HBV is highest amongst people with particular lifestyle or occupational risks, such as midwives and student midwives. Vaccination is recommended for healthcare workers who might have direct contact with patients' blood, blood-stained body fluids or tissues. Health workers are recommended to have one vaccine booster 5 years after the primary vaccination (PHE 2017) and to follow universal precautions for reducing the risk of infection (Table 8.2).

Women with hepatitis B should have their care referred to and managed by a multi-disciplinary team, including a hepatologist, gastroenterologist or infectious diseases specialist. Consultations should preferably take place within 6 weeks of a seropositive result. As part of the consultation, it is important that women are able to discuss notification of the infection, testing for their close contacts and measures to limit the spread of infection (DH 2011). Named antenatal screening midwives or

Table 8.1: **A summary of the results and implications of serum markers for HBV**

Serum marker	Result	Implication
HBsAg	Negative	Susceptible to infection; consider vaccination
Anti-HBc	Negative	
Anti-HBs	Negative	
HBsAg	Negative	Natural immunity
Anti-HBc	Positive	
Anti-HBs	Positive	
HBsAg	Negative	Immune response to vaccine
Anti-HBc	Negative	
Anti-HBs	Positive	
HBsAg	Positive	Acute HBV infection
Anti-HBc	Positive	
IgM anti-HBc	Positive	
Anti-HBs	Negative	
HBsAg	Positive	Chronic HBV infection
Anti-HBc	Positive	
IgM anti-HBc	Negative	
Anti-HBs	Negative	
HBsAg	Negative	Possible implications
Anti-HBc	Positive	• Infection is resolved
Anti-HBs	Negative	• False-positive anti-HBc – susceptible
		• 'Low-level' chronic infection
		• Resolving acute infection

Created from data from (CDC 2018a)

coordinators are normally responsible for managing screening and immunization programmes, as well as ensuring effective multi-disciplinary communication, which should include a neonatal alert (DH 2011).

Mother-to-child-transmission (MTCT) of HBV

Perinatal transmission between mother and baby can be reduced by offering routine serological HBV screening to pregnant women as part of the Infectious Diseases in Pregnancy Screening (IDPS) Programme (PHE 2016) and offering appropriate and effective postnatal interventions, to include selective neonatal immunization (PHE 2017). Such interventions can reduce mother-to-baby transmission by about 90%, and discussions with the woman about hepatitis B screening and vaccination should emphasize the potential benefits for her baby (DH 2011). PHE (2017) recommends commencement of the neonatal immunization programme within 24 hours of birth and further immunizations at 4

Table 8.2: Reducing the risk of occupational exposure to bloodborne infection (BBV)

Assess the risk of exposure.

Eliminate or control the risk using safe systems of work (adhering to health and safety policies) and personal protective equipment (PPE).

Minimize risk of exposure to blood products and BBV.

Avoid contact with blood or bodily fluids.

Take all necessary precautions to prevent puncture wounds, cuts and abrasions in the presence of blood and body fluids.

Avoid using sharps (e.g. needles, metal) if possible; take care in handling sharps where unavoidable; discard sharp instruments directly into the approved sharps container immediately after and at the point of use.

Protect all exposed skin lesions with waterproof dressings and/or gloves.

Use PPE, such as goggles, masks, waterproof clothing, plastic apron, rubber boots or overshoes, when contamination is possible. Careful and thorough hygiene precautions, such as handwashing before and after each patient contact and glove use; avoid hand-to-mouth/eye contact.

Manage surface contamination by containing body fluids and decontamination.

Safe disposal of all contaminated waste, referring to relevant guidance.

Adapted from Health & Safety Executive (n.d.)

and 8 weeks and 1 year. Babies who are born to mothers who are highly infectious should receive both active (vaccine) and passive (immunoglobulin) protection. Babies who are born preterm should have immunizations at the relevant chronological age and may benefit from maternal antenatal steroid therapy. Since 2017, HBV immunization is included in the routine childhood immunization programme (PHE 2017). Hepatitis immunoglobulin (HBIG) is sourced from the plasma of immunized and screened donors and provides passive immunity. It can provide temporary but immediate protection after contact with HBV-infected blood until the hepatitis B vaccine, which is ideally given within 24 hours, becomes effective (PHE 2017).

Activity

What are the potential barriers to an effective HBV screening and immunization programme? What possible solutions are available to midwives and other service providers?

Hepatitis C

HCV is a slow, progressive and unpredictable disease whose impact can vary from minimal symptoms to terminal liver failure or liver carcinoma. HCV is bloodborne, placing people at risk if they are exposed to another person's blood, and transmission is most commonly (60%) associated with intravenous drug use (Silasi et al 2015). Vertical transmission from mother to fetus occurs in around 6% of mothers with chronic HCV and increases to 14% to 17% for mothers who are also infected with HIV or who have prolonged rupture of membranes. Approximately 25% to 50% of people spontaneously clear the virus within 6 months (National Institute for Health and Care Excellence (NICE) 2016). NICE (2008) does not recommend routine screening for HCV due to limited evidence of clinical effectiveness and cost-effectiveness.

Mother-to-child-transmission of HCV

Whilst vertical transmission cannot be prevented, awareness of a pregnant woman's positive HCV status may enable midwives to reduce risks to the fetus by avoiding the use of fetal scalp electrodes or ensuring that the baby's skin is thoroughly cleaned before any injections or blood sampling (Bothamley & Boyle 2015). Babies born to infected mothers are more likely to have a lower birth weight, be born preterm or have adverse neurological outcomes (Salemi et al 2014); their HCV status can be determined through serological testing (NICE 2016). Breastfeeding is not known to pose a risk to babies (Silasi et al 2015). Since there is no HCV immunization and midwives can be exposed to the blood of childbearing women whose HCV status is unknown, HCV poses a significant risk, and following universal safety precautions is imperative.

Activity

Access the British Liver Trust website (*https://www.britishlivertrust. org.uk/*) to find groups who support people with liver conditions in your area.

Human immunodeficiency virus

HIV is a retrovirus which, if untreated, leads to suppressed immunity for the infected person and eventually AIDS (PHE 2016). This process can take months or years, with an average of 11 years (CDC 2015a). CD4 cells (T-helper cells) are white blood cells which play an important role in immunity and antibody production: normal levels are 500 to 1500 cells/ml blood. HIV invades and destroys CD4 cells, reducing serum levels and lowering immunity, and if the infection is untreated, the infected person becomes vulnerable to other infections and HIV-related cancers (PHE 2016). A CD4 count of <350 cells/ml increases opportunistic infections, and CD4 <200 cells/ml makes the host particularly vulnerable (Bothamley & Boyle 2015). During the acute stage after initial infection, concentrations of the virus are elevated, causing a highly infectious condition.

Transmission of HIV

HIV is present in an infected person's bodily fluids and can be transmitted via unprotected sexual intercourse, direct contact with infected blood, sharing infected needles, transplacentally from mother to fetus or in breast milk (PHE 2016). Within a few weeks of becoming infected 50% to 90% of infected people present with vague symptoms such as fever, enlarged lymph glands, malaise and skin rashes. However, antibody tests in early stages may be negative (CDC 2015a) and may need to be repeated if symptoms present later or there are ongoing risks (Bothamley & Boyle 2015). HIV tests assist in making a swift diagnosis so that treatment can commence. Management aims to restrict the spread of infection and improve life expectancy and quality, whilst considering relative care costs. Antiretroviral therapy (ART) can reduce transmission of the infection, limit the severity of acute illness, reduce viral replication and mutation and maintain immune processes (CDC 2015a).

Mother-to-child-transmission of HIV

Mother-to-child transmission (MTCT) of HIV has been significantly reduced in the UK as a consequence of routine antenatal screening, ART and avoidance of breastfeeding. The rate of MTCT in untreated mothers is around 25%, but early diagnosis and management can reduce this to less than 0.5% (PHE 2016). Mothers with a high VL and low CD4 count have an increased chance of MTCT (Bothamley & Boyle 2015). By 2010, 98% of pregnant women with HIV in the UK received ART antenatally, reducing their risk of MTCT. As a consequence, the numbers of women having vaginal births more than doubled and elective caesarean sections reduced by half from 2006 to 2010 (British HIV Association (BHIVA) 2014).

Screening

Initial screening for HIV is offered at the woman's pregnancy booking and involves early pregnancy serological testing for HIV-1 antibodies, HIV-1 p24 antigen and HIV-2 antibodies (PHE 2016). Where women decline early screening or are viewed as being at high risk of infection, testing should be re-offered at 28 weeks' gestation (BHIVA 2014) and before 36 weeks (CDC 2015a). Screening for HIV is part of the role of the midwife, who must ensure that women have a good understanding of the screening process and implications of a positive result before undertaking the blood sampling. Discussions should include the potential benefits of diagnosing HIV, such as reducing MTCT and improving the mother's own health. Women who are diagnosed with HIV infection should be offered screening for HBV, syphilis and other sexually transmitted infections (STIs) due to the increased incidence of co-infections (BHIVA 2014; CDC 2015a). In addition, midwives can offer guidance about safe sex and avoiding high-risk activities. The majority of HIV-positive pregnant women in the UK are of sub-Saharan Africa origin (BHIVA 2014). Pregnancy does not appear to affect the course of HIV infection (Silasi et al 2015), and during pregnancy, ultrasound screening is offered as per routine care. The preferred methods of screening for Down's syndrome are pregnancy-associated plasma protein A (PAPP-A) and nuchal fold translucency measurements, which are unaffected by HIV or antiretroviral drugs (BHIVA 2014).

Treatment for HIV

Drug therapy for HIV is normally a combination of three drugs known as *highly active antiretroviral therapy (HAART)*. The use of triple antiretroviral drugs is most effective in reducing MTCT (Siegfried et al 2011), and using combined drugs helps avoid drug resistance, moderates side effects and minimizes the required dose of each drug to lessen toxicity. Side effects from the drugs, such as gastrointestinal upset, can be similar to pregnancy conditions and should be investigated to avoid missing co-existing complications (Bothamley & Boyle 2015). Treatment is determined by serological assessments and co-existing health issues, such as hepatitis or tuberculosis. HAART is usually commenced before 24 weeks' gestation if the woman is not already receiving treatment, or immediately if booking is after this gestation (BHIVA 2014).

The aim of treatment is to achieve a VL of <50 copies/ml blood by 36 weeks' gestation, when the multi-disciplinary team will discuss plans for labour and birth with the woman. If the fetus is presenting by the breech at 36 weeks, the VL is <50 copies/ml and there are no other complications, external cephalic version can be offered (BHIVA 2014). The recommended mode of birth is dependent on VL, and Table 8.3 provides an overview of considerations for management during labour and birth.

Care of the neonate

To reduce the risk of neonatal transmission through maternal blood and secretions, the baby can be towel dried and washed immediately after birth. The use of alcohol wipes for cleaning specific sites of injections or blood testing contributes to minimizing transmission risks (Bothamley & Boyle 2015). If the mother's VL is >50 copies/ml, the baby will be

Table 8.3: **Considerations for labour and birth**

- VL <50 copies/ml – plan for vaginal birth.
- VL 50–399 copies/ml – consider planned caesarean section, whilst taking into account the VL trajectory, the length of time of ART, obstetric considerations and the woman's views.
- VL >400 copies/ml – planned caesarean section is recommended.
- ART is continued during labour and may include an intravenous infusion of zidovudine, particularly for women who are untreated, their VL is unknown or is >100,000 copies/ml, there is prolonged rupture of membranes or planned caesarean section.
- MTCT is likely to be low following fetal scalp sampling or fetal scalp electrode use where the VL <50 copies/ml.
- Links between MTCT and instrumental birth, amniotomy and episiotomy have not been established; avoiding these procedures is not evidence based. If instrumental birth is indicated, forceps are recommended, as this is considered less traumatic for the baby.
- Universal precautions should be used to reduce the risk posed to carers in labour and birth; midwives are at particularly high risk of exposure to HIV due to repeated and unexpected exposure to large volumes of blood.

Based on BHIVA (2014)

commenced on post-exposure prophylaxis (PEP) ART. All babies born to mothers with HIV should be tested at birth, at 6 and 12 weeks and again at 18 months (BHIVA 2014). They should receive coordinated care from a specialist multi-disciplinary team; specialist input may be particularly pertinent for preterm babies who may be unable to tolerate oral drugs.

Feeding issues

HIV-positive mothers in the UK are encouraged to exclusively formula feed their babies, regardless of their compliance with treatment, serological status or newborn PEP. Midwives can discuss lactation suppression during the antenatal period. When mothers choose to breastfeed against medical advice, their adherence to ART and serological markers are closely monitored, alongside monthly monitoring and diagnostic testing of the baby (PHE 2016). Where mothers with a detectable VL choose to breastfeed their baby, this is a safeguarding issue on account of the high risk of transmission (BHIVA 2014). After birth, midwives can remind women with HIV of the importance of taking care of themselves as well as their baby and discuss pre-conception care for future pregnancies.

Psychosocial issues

Women who are diagnosed with HIV during pregnancy can feel vulnerable. They may have little time to process information relating to important decisions and to build trust in health professionals. Whilst disclosure of their HIV diagnosis to partners or close family is encouraged, fears about stigmatization can make women reluctant (Kontomanolis et al 2017). Some women fear that taking medications and not breastfeeding might act as 'disclosure by association' (BHIVA 2014:54), and midwives can help women provide alternative explanations for such actions. Confidentiality is vital, although where women are reluctant to disclose to partners, this can place midwives in a difficult ethical and potentially legal position. Breaking confidentiality is considered to be a last resort (BHIVA 2014; Nursing and Midwifery Council (NMC) 2015).

Activity

For more information about your responsibility for protecting yourself and others from exposure to bloodborne infection, read the guidance from the Health and Safety Executive (*http://www.hse.gov.uk/biosafety/diseases/bbv.pdf*).

Syphilis

Syphilis is caused by the *Treponema pallidum* bacterium. It is a disease that is transmitted sexually or from mother to fetus (congenital syphilis) (CDC 2018b; PHE 2016). The average incubation period is around 21 days, when the first symptoms occur, but it is a disease of several stages. The primary stage presents as a painless sore (chancre) at the infection site. This lasts for 3 to 6 weeks, can remain unnoticed and normally heals spontaneously. Without treatment the infection progresses to a second stage with sores on mucous membranes and skin rashes, typically on the palms of the hands and soles of the feet. Other symptoms include condyloma lata (raised lesions in the mouth or groin), pyrexia, aches, weight loss and tiredness (CDC 2018b). If allowed to progress, syphilis then undergoes a symptomless period of latency, which can last several years. Tertiary syphilis can occur 10 to 30 years after the primary infection; it affects multiple organs and can be fatal.

Screening for syphilis

Antenatal screening as part of the IDPP aims to reduce the risk of congenital syphilis and involves serological testing for antibodies to *T. pallidum* (PHE 2016). In very early infections these antibodies may be undeveloped, so the infection may be missed. Confirmatory testing provides a strong indication of past or present infection but cannot differentiate. Referral to a specialist in genitourinary medicine is important (PHE 2016); pregnant women with active syphilis or who were not treated for a prior infection should be offered treatment with a single dose of benzyl penicillin and referred to fetal medicine.

Pregnancy outcome

Around 40% of pregnant women with untreated syphilis will experience perinatal death of their baby. Babies who survive may be born prematurely or have a low birth weight; there may be signs of congenital syphilis, such as enlarged liver and spleen, rhinitis jaundice or a skin rash (CDC 2018b). Initially they can appear symptom-free, but from around 2 years of age may develop bony abnormalities, hepatosplenomegaly, glomerulonephritis or neurological damage (Bothamley & Boyle 2015). Therefore, babies of mothers with syphilis require careful assessment and syphilis serology testing with neonatal and paediatric follow-up (CDC 2018b; PHE 2016).

Influenza (flu)

Haemophilus influenza virus is transmitted via droplets and can produce symptoms such as cough, pyrexia, malaise, headache, sore throat and tachycardia (Silasi et al 2015). Invasive infection can cause serious illness, and changes in a pregnant woman's immunity make her particularly vulnerable to severe illness for herself (such as meningitis and pneumonia) and her fetus (for instance, neural tube defects, premature birth and low birth weight) (PHE 2013). Women with underlying health conditions such as asthma are at even greater risk (Silasi et al 2015). If pregnant women develop flu, they should be carefully observed, offered anti-viral treatment as soon as possible (within 48 hours of developing symptoms) and encouraged to adopt cooling strategies such as taking paracetamol. Each NHS trust will have a local strategy for caring for patients with a positive flu diagnosis, and these must be carefully followed for the protection of women, other patients and staff.

Vaccination

During 2009–2011, 27 indirect maternal deaths due to influenza were reported in the UK; half of these deaths might have been prevented through vaccination (Churchill et al 2014). Vaccinating all pregnant women annually against flu is now a public health priority (PHE 2015) and World Health Organization (2018) recommendation. Flu vaccines given in pregnancy are inactivated; they do not contain live organisms and cannot cause flu. However, there may be discomfort at the injection site, and some women experience a brief episode of feeling unwell as their immune responses activate. Flu vaccination can be given at any time during pregnancy, although earlier vaccination provides longer pregnancy protection. Vaccination protects the mother and baby against flu during and after pregnancy for up to 6 months; it is not known to be harmful during pregnancy or breastfeeding (PHE 2015). Midwives are responsible for informing all pregnant women about the dangers of flu in pregnancy, the potential benefits of vaccination and local arrangements for providing this.

Group B Streptococcus

Group B streptococcus (GBS) is a bacterium that is carried in the vagina or rectum of 20% to 24% of women in the UK. Most carriers will be symptomless, although GBS can be particularly harmful to some babies around the time of birth, causing sepsis, pneumonia or meningitis (Royal College of Obstetricians and Gynaecologists and Group B Strep Support (RCOG & GBSS) 2017). More rarely, GBS infection is associated with miscarriage, premature birth or stillbirth (UK National Screening Committee (UKNSC) 2017). GBS can be detected by vaginal or rectal swabs or urine testing. Screening is not routine in the UK. The rationale for this is that most babies born to women with GBS will be unaffected, screening does not predict which babies will be affected, screening is recommended at around 35 to 37 weeks which would be too late for babies born prematurely, there is a risk of false-negative results and many women would be unnecessarily treated with antibiotics (RCOG & GBSS 2017; UKNSC 2017). There is currently no immunization for women against GBS in the UK, although information about GBS should be provided (RCOG 2017).

Testing women for GBS

Women who were diagnosed with GBS in a previous pregnancy have a 50% chance of recurrence and should be offered testing at 35 to 37 weeks' gestation, with a positive result indicating a risk of neonatal GBS infection of around 1 in 400, or 1 in 5000 for a negative result. Intrapartum antibiotics will be offered to these women and to women who have had a previous baby with early-onset GBS infection, regardless of bacteriological testing. Women whose urine tests positive for GBS should receive treatment at the time of diagnosis and intrapartum antibiotics (RCOG 2017). Pre-labour rupture of membranes after 37 weeks' gestation is an indication for induction of labour with antibiotic cover to reduce the window for transmission. The presence of GBS is not a contraindication for membrane sweeping or for use of a birthing pool. The administration of benzylpenicillin for women having a caesarean section will be reviewed individually and will depend on factors such as the gestation, indication for caesarean section and rupture of membranes. Allergies to penicillin can cause anaphylactic shock; alternative anti-microbials can be given where allergies are known (CDC 2015b; RCOG 2017; RCOG & GBSS 2017).

Neonatal GBS infection

GBS infection in the first week of life is known as *early-onset GBS infection (EOGBS)*; most affected babies develop signs within the first 12 hours (UKNSC 2017). It affects around 1 in 1750 babies and is the most common cause of severe early-onset neonatal infection (RCOG 2017). Other causes of neonatal sepsis include *Escherichia coli, Staphylococcus aureus, Enterococcus, Listeria monocytogenes, Klebsiella* and *Pseudomonas* (Voller & Myers 2016). Treatment using intrapartum antibiotics (normally benzylpenicillin) for women with GBS has reduced the incidence of EOGBS by 87% (Voller & Myers 2016). However, neonatal GBS is still a significant cause for concern since it is associated with 5.2% mortality and 7.4% long-term morbidity rates (RCOG & GBSS 2017). Factors increasing the risk of neonatal GBS include prematurity, previous baby affected by GBS, intrapartum infection or pyrexia, evidence of GBS infection (positive urine or vaginal and ano-rectal microbiology) and rupture of membranes over 24 hours (RCOG & GBSS 2017).

If a woman with GBS declines intrapartum antibiotics or has received antibiotics less than 4 hours before birth, her baby should be monitored carefully for 12 hours for signs of infection, such as unstable temperature, lethargy or irritability, respiratory changes, poor feeding, distended abdomen, jaundice and tachycardia (Voller & Myers 2016). Where neonatal infection is suspected, a neonatal review is vital, and investigations such as blood or cerebrospinal fluid microbiology will be performed to confirm or exclude the diagnosis and antibiotic treatment commenced urgently. GBS is not an indication to discourage breastfeeding (RCOG 2017).

Look back on the trigger scenario.

Sara and Mike are delighted when a pregnancy test confirms that Sara is pregnant with their second baby. Despite feeling excited, Sara is also worried. She gave birth to George at 34 weeks' gestation, and he required treatment on the neonatal unit for an infection. That was a worrying time for the couple, and Sara blamed herself for George's illness. As she makes a note of the first appointment with her midwife, she wonders what she can do to prevent a similar situation occurring this time.

Now that you are familiar with how these infections relate to childbearing, you should have insight into how the scenario relates to the evidence. The jigsaw model will now be used to explore the trigger scenario in more depth.

Effective communication

Effective communication between women and midwives is a two-way process, involving verbal and non-verbal information-sharing. Midwives have a responsibility to ensure that childbearing women are able to make informed choices relating to their own and their baby's health. Questions that arise from this scenario might include: How can the midwife ensure that Sara has sufficient understanding and support to make an informed choice about screening, diagnostic testing and immunization against infectious diseases in pregnancy? What questions might the midwife have regarding Sara's previous experience? How could non-verbal communication skills impact on the interactions between Sara and her midwife?

Woman-centred care

Screening and treatment programmes should be adapted to meet the individual physical, psychosocial and emotional needs of women and their families. Questions that arise from the scenario might include: How can midwives support childbearing women, such as Sara, with the psychosocial and emotional issues associated with the diagnosis of infectious diseases? What does Sara know already about reducing the risk of pregnancy-related infections? Were Sara and Mike given the opportunity to discuss the reasons for George's illness and whether this might occur in a subsequent pregnancy?

Using best evidence

Keeping up to date with the best available evidence helps midwives ensure that they are using the most appropriate skills and knowledge in their practice to prevent, detect or treat infections. Questions that arise from the scenario might include: What does the most recent antenatal screening programme recommend for reducing infectious diseases in pregnancy? What advice can midwives give to women to reduce the risk of MTCT of infections? Why is universal screening for GBS offered in some other developed countries but not in the UK?

Professional and legal issues

Midwives must always practise within the law, uphold their professional guidelines and be accountable for their decisions. Questions that arise from the scenario might include: How can midwives maintain confidentiality whilst ensuring that they meet their professional and legal requirements for documentation and information-sharing? How can midwives demonstrate the actions they have or have not taken? What actions can a midwife take if women make decisions which deviate from guidance? How can midwives ensure that they have gained informed consent for procedures involving women?

Team working

Women who have one of the previously discussed infections will have additional care needs. Whilst midwives are responsible for involving appropriate professionals in the care of women with additional or complex needs, they are also responsible for coordinating and involving women in decisions about their care. Questions that midwives might consider include: In what ways could involving women and the multi-disciplinary team in developing guidelines for preventing, detecting and managing infectious diseases in pregnancy lead to better outcomes? What strategies could enhance effective continuity of carer and reduce delays in the treatment and diagnosis of infectious diseases for childbearing women?

Clinical dexterity

In this scenario, the midwife is likely to take blood samples from Sara as part of the screening for infectious diseases programme. She may need to obtain urine, vaginal or rectal swabs. Questions that arise from the scenario might include: How has the midwife developed phlebotomy skills, and are any measures in place to audit midwives' practices?

If the midwife was unable to obtain the required sample, what measures are in place for ensuring that this does not get missed? What facilities are there in the community for taking and transporting blood, urine or other specimens?

Models of care

There are various models of midwifery care, including case loading, team midwifery and a more traditional approach whereby women are supported in the community by a community midwife and for their birth by hospital or birth centre midwives. Questions that arise from this scenario might include: How can Sara build a trusting relationship with the midwife who supports her labour and birth if they have not met previously? If there is a chance that Sara's baby might need to be treated for an infection, what care provisions are available to keep Sara and her baby together? How might separation of Sara and her newborn affect their early relationship?

Safe environment

Infections can be transmitted through direct or indirect contact. Maintaining a safe environment is essential in reducing the risk of healthcare-related infections for service users and staff. Questions that arise from the scenario might include: Why is it important for midwives to maintain their personal health in relation to their practice? What programmes are in place to reduce the risks of bloodborne infections for midwives and student midwives? What precautions can midwives take to minimize their risk of work-related infections? What actions should be taken if the midwife observes or is asked to participate in unsafe practices?

Promotes health

Promoting wellbeing and preventing ill health are key responsibilities of the midwife and, in relation to the prevention and management of infections in pregnancy, involve safe ways of working, information-sharing, screening and diagnostic and treatment programmes. Issues that might arise in relation to Sara include: How might Sara's lifestyle affect her and her baby's vulnerability to infection? What considerations might the midwife discuss with Sara to promote her health during pregnancy? How can the midwife work with Sara and Mike to promote their family's health in the longer term?

Further scenarios

The following scenarios enable you to consider how specific situations influence the care the midwife provides. Use the jigsaw model to explore the issues raised in the scenarios.

Amina is 23 and moved to England from sub-Saharan Africa several months ago. English is Amina's second language. She meets with her community midwife at 26 weeks' gestation for a booking appointment. Her sister-in-law attends the appointment with her.

Women who are new to the UK may be unaware of the maternity care available to them or how to access this; they can therefore miss out on important information, investigations and aspects of care. Language barriers can inhibit or distort information-sharing and understanding for both the midwife and the woman, and whilst family members or friends might be conversant in both languages, they may be unable to translate medical terminology, and the midwife has no way of confirming the accuracy or completeness of what is being said. Furthermore, the presence of family members may inhibit disclosure about sensitive issues.

Questions that could be asked are:
1. To what extent is Amina's use of the English language sufficient for her to understand the questions and information-sharing that will take place during the booking appointment?
2. How can the midwife ensure that her communication with Amina is effective?
3. Why might Amina have presented for midwifery care at this stage of pregnancy?
4. In what ways might Amina's background affect her risk of having or developing infectious diseases?
5. How can the midwife preserve Amina's privacy, dignity and confidentiality during this appointment?

James is a second-year student midwife and has just started a placement with a community midwife. He has completed his phlebotomy skills training and is eager to practise his technique. After gaining consent from the pregnant woman and under the supervision of Janine, his mentor, he successfully draws a blood sample, but as James moves to discard the needle and syringe, he accidentally pricks his finger with the used needle.

Practice point

Midwives have a joint responsibility with their employers to protect the health and safety of themselves, their colleagues and the people in their care. Employers have a duty to provide safe working conditions and policies to reduce the potential for harm. Employees are responsible for adhering to health and safety policies and for reporting adverse incidents in a timely manner.

Questions that could be asked are:
1. What are the potential risks for James in this situation?
2. How might this needle-stick injury have been avoided?
3. What actions should now be taken by James and his mentor and in what timescale?
4. How will this incident be documented?
5. What measures are in place for healthcare workers such as midwives and student midwives to reduce the risk of acquiring infectious diseases in the course of their practice?

Conclusion

This chapter has provided an overview of some of the infections in pregnancy, childbirth and the postnatal period that pose a significant threat to the mother, her baby and her family and those providing their care. Midwives are responsible for communicating effectively with women to share information; assess women's likelihood of having or acquiring infections; and provide screening, appropriate treatment and support. Furthermore, having a sound evidence base and skills relating to the identification of infection and reducing the spread of infection, as well as effective team working, enable midwives to protect the safety of the women and babies in their care and their personal and colleagues' safety, and contributes to reducing infection-related maternal and perinatal mortality and morbidity.

Resources

Advisory Committee on Dangerous Pathogens Protection against blood-borne infections in the workplace: HIV and Hepatitis: http://www.hse.gov.uk/biosafety/diseases/bbv.pdf

British Liver Trust: https://www.britishlivertrust.org.uk/

Centers for Disease Control and Prevention (CDC), 2017. Pregnant women & influenza (flu). Available at: https://www.cdc.gov/flu/protect/vaccine/pregnant.htm.

NHS Infection. Prevention. Control.: https://www.infectionpreventioncontrol.co.uk/healthcare-professionals/

Sexwise (information from the Family Planning Association (FPA) for the National Health Promotion Programme for Sexual Health and Reproductive Health): https://sexwise.fpa.org.uk/

Terrence Higgins Trust (HIV and sexual health charity): https://www.tht.org.uk/

References

Bothamley, J., Boyle, M., 2015. Infections Affecting Pregnancy and Childbirth. Radcliffe Publishing, London.

British HIV Association (BHIVA), 2014. British HIV Association guidelines for the management of HIV infection in pregnant women 2012 (2014 Interim Review). Available at: http://www.bhiva.org/documents/Guidelines/Pregnancy/2012/BHIVA-Pregnancy-guidelines-update-2014.pdf.

Centers for Disease Control and Prevention (CDC), 2015a. HIV Infection: Detection, Counseling, and Referral. Available at: https://www.cdc.gov/std/tg2015/hiv.htm.

Centers for Disease Control and Prevention (CDC), 2015b. Sexually Transmitted Diseases Treatment Guidelines. Available at: https://www.cdc.gov/std/tg2015/tg-2015-print.pdf.

Centers for Disease Control and Prevention (CDC), 2018a. Viral Hepatitis. Available at: http://www.cdc.gov/hepatitis/hbv/hbvfaq.htm#general.

Centers for Disease Control and Prevention (CDC), 2018b. Sex. Transm. Dis. Available at: https://www.cdc.gov/std/default.htm.

Churchill, D., Rodger, A., Clift, J., Tuffnell, D., on behalf of the MBRRACE-UK sepsis chapter writing group, 2014. Think sepsis. In: Knight, M., Kenyon, S., Brocklehurst, P., et al. on behalf of MBRRACEUK (Eds.), Saving Lives, Improving Mothers' Care – Lessons Learned to Inform Future Maternity Care From the UK and Ireland Confidential Enquiries Into Maternal Deaths and Morbidity 2009–12. National Perinatal Epidemiology Unit, University of Oxford, Oxford, pp. 27–43.

Department of Health and Social Care, 2011. Hepatitis B antenatal screening and newborn immunisation programme: Best practice guidance. Available at: https://www.gov.uk/government/publications/hepatitis-b-antenatal-screening-and-newborn-immunisation-programme-best-practice-guidance.

Draper, E.S., Gallimore, I.D., Kurinczuk, J.J., et al. on behalf of the MBRRACE-UK Collaboration, 2018. MBRRACE-UK Perinatal Mortality Surveillance Report, UK Perinatal Deaths for Births from January to December 2016. Leicester: The Infant Mortality and Morbidity Studies, Department of Health Sciences, University of Leicester.

Eke, A.C., Eleje, G.U., Eke, U.A., et al., 2017. Hepatitis B immunoglobulin during pregnancy for prevention of mother-to-child transmission of hepatitis B virus. Cochrane Database Syst. Rev. (2), CD008545, doi:10.1002/14651858.CD008545.pub2.

Health and Safety Executive Advisory Committee on Dangerous Pathogens, (n.d.). Protection against blood-borne infections in the workplace: HIV and Hepatitis. Available at: http://www.hse.gov.uk/biosafety/diseases/bbv.pdf.

Knight, M., Nair, M., Tuffnell, D., et al. on behalf of MBRRACE-UK (Eds.), 2017. Saving Lives, Improving Mothers' Care – Lessons Learned to Inform Maternity Care From the UK and Ireland Confidential Enquiries Into Maternal Deaths and Morbidity 2013–15. National Perinatal Epidemiology Unit, University of Oxford, Oxford.

Kontomanolis, E.N., Michalopoulos, S., Gkasdaris, G., Fasoulakis, Z., 2017. The social stigma of HIV-AIDS: society's role. HIV/AIDS – Research and Palliative Care 9, 111–118. doi:10.2147/HIV.S129992.

Krajden, M., McNabb, G., Petric, M., 2005. The laboratory diagnosis of hepatitis B virus. Canadian Journal of Infectious Diseases and Medical Microbiology. 16 (2), 65–72. Available at: https://www.ncbi.nlm.nih.gov/pmc/articles/PMC2095015/.

National Institute for Health and Care Excellence (NICE), 2008. Antenatal care for uncomplicated pregnancies. Available at: https://www.nice.org.uk/Guidance/CG62.

National Institute for Health and Care Excellence (NICE), 2016. Clinical knowledge summary: Hepatitis C. Available at: https://cks.nice.org.uk/hepatitis-c#!topicsummary.

Nursing and Midwifery Council, 2015. The Code: Professional standards of practice and behaviour for nurses and midwives. Available at: https://www.nmc.org.uk/globalassets/sitedocuments/nmc-publications/nmc-code.pdf.

Public Health England, 2013. The Green Book: Immunisation against infectious disease. Available at: https://www.gov.uk/government/collections/immunisation-against-infectious-disease-the-green-book – Information adapted under Open Government Licence v3.0 https://www.nationalarchives.gov.uk/doc/open-government-licence/version/3/.

Public Health England, 2015. Influenza vaccination in pregnancy: information for healthcare professionals. Available at: https://www.gov.uk/government/uploads/system/uploads/attachment_data/file/393974/Influenza_vaccination_in_pregnancy_factsheet_v15_CT__2_.pdf.

Public Health England, 2016. NHS Infectious Diseases in Pregnancy Screening (IDPS) Programme Handbook 2016-2017. Available at: https://www.gov.uk/topic/population-screening-programmes/infectious-diseases-in-pregnancy.

Public Health England, 2017. The Green Book: Immunisation against infectious disease. Chapter 18. Hepatitis B. Available at: https://www.gov.uk/government/collections/immunisation-against-infectious-disease-the-green-book – Information adapted under Open Government Licence v3.0 https://www.nationalarchives.gov.uk/doc/open-government-licence/version/3/.

Royal College of Obstetricians and Gynaecologists (RCOG), 2017. Prevention of early onset Group B Streptococcal disease: Greentop Guideline No.36 (3rd Ed.). Available at: https://obgyn.onlinelibrary.wiley.com/doi/full/10.1111/1471-0528.14821.

Royal College of Obstetricians and Gynaecologists and Group B Strep Support (GBSS), 2017. Group B Streptococcus (GBS) in pregnancy and newborn babies. Available at: https://gbss.org.uk/wp-content/uploads/2018/01/2017-Joint-RCOG-GBSS-PIL_final.pdf.

Salemi, J.L., Whiteman, V.E., August, E.M., et al., 2014. Maternal hepatitis B and hepatitis C infection and neonatal neurological outcomes. J. Viral Hepat. 21 (11), e144–e153. doi:10.1111/jvh.12250.

Siegfried, N., van der Merwe, L., Brocklehurst, P., Sint, T.T., 2011. Antiretrovirals for reducing the risk of mother-to-child transmission of HIV infection. Cochrane Database Syst. Rev. (7), CD003510, doi:10.1002/14651858. CD003510.pub3.

Silasi, M., Cardenas, I., Kwon, J.Y., et al., 2015. Viral infections during pregnancy. Am. J. Reprod. Immunol. 73 (3), 199–213. doi:10.1111/aji.12355.

UK National Screening Committee, 2017. The UK NSC Recommendation on Group B Streptococcus Screening in Pregnancy. Available at: https://legacyscreening.phe.org.uk/groupbstreptococcus.

Voller, S.M.B., Myers, P.J., 2016. Neonatal sepsis. Clinical Pediatric Emergency Medicine 17 (2), 129–133. doi:10.1016/j.cpem.2016.03.006.

World Health Organisation (WHO), 2018. Influenza (seasonal). Available at: http://www.who.int/en/news-room/fact-sheets/detail/influenza-(seasonal).

CHAPTER 9

Neurological conditions

TRIGGER SCENARIO

Julie and her partner, Joe, are waiting in the hospital antenatal clinic for their detailed scan. Julie was diagnosed with epilepsy when she was 6 years old and has been under the care of a neurologist throughout her childhood. She turns to Joe and says, 'Do you think they will be able to tell if our baby has been damaged by that fit I had last week?'

Introduction

Becoming pregnant and becoming a parent is a significant event in any woman's life. When this incredible event is combined with a pre-existing neurological disease, antenatal, intrapartum and postnatal care need careful consideration to ensure that a safe and satisfying outcome is achieved for all. It is therefore important that the midwife is able to care for women in partnership with her, acknowledging the unique insight the woman and her family may already have into her condition.

There are myriad neurological conditions, and many of these are so rare that often midwives can go through their career never having cared for anyone with that particular condition. Other conditions, such as epilepsy, are more common but vary in their origin and/or severity. Thus the focus of this chapter is to describe those conditions that the midwife is most likely to encounter and to provide the skills for recognizing the signs and symptoms of neurological disorders that may develop during pregnancy. In addition, some potential pregnancy- and birth-related neurological deficits will be described.

Context

When considering neurological conditions, we need to differentiate between those that are affected by pregnancy, those that develop in pregnancy and those that are a consequence of labour and birth. When women have a pre-existing condition, especially when drug therapy is a key component of its management, women of childbearing age should be advised to seek pre-conceptual care from their neurologist.

Neurological examination

A detailed clinical examination of the woman's neurological wellbeing is indicated for women who are known to have a pre-existing neurological condition and become pregnant and those who develop symptoms in pregnancy. Whether a full examination is conducted will depend on whether the symptoms are new, severe and/or potentially life threatening, for example, sudden loss of consciousness.

Learning from maternal mortality reports, it is suggested that neurological examination is mandatory for all new-onset headaches, particularly those with focal symptoms, and this should include assessment for neck stiffness (Knight et al 2014) and fundoscopy (Knight et al 2015). Red flag headache symptoms (Box 9.1) were further highlighted in a subsequent maternal mortality report (Knight et al 2017), and presentation of these should precipitate urgent action.

Focal neurological signs or deficits

These result from impairments of brain, spine or nerve function that affect a specific region of the body. These focal signs include changes in:

+ Speech
+ Hearing
+ Vision
+ Smell
+ Sensation, pain and temperature
+ Reflexes
+ Balance, coordination and gait
+ Memory, processing, behaviour and emotions
+ Muscle power, rigidity, tone and symmetry

Activity

What is meant by the term *meningism*? What is the significance of neck stiffness when associated with headache and fever?

Box 9.1 Red flag headache symptoms

- Headache of sudden onset, described as the 'worst ever'
- Headaches with additional symptoms not usually experienced: neck stiffness, fever, weakness, double vision, drowsiness, seizures
- A headache that takes longer to resolve than usual or persists longer than 48 hours

From (Knight et al 2017:35)

Consciousness

If the patient is unconscious, it is essential that principles of caring for the collapsed woman be implemented immediately. This includes ensuring that help is on its way, her airway is patent and assessing her breathing and cardiac status (see Volume 6, Chapter 1 in the *Midwifery Essentials* series).

It is then essential that a potential cause is identified, and this would include exploring:

+ If the woman has taken any drugs that may have impacted on her consciousness level
+ Biochemical status, e.g. electrolyte imbalance, hypoglycaemia
+ Potential status epilepticus
+ Injury or electrocution

Observations

Glasgow Coma Scale

Developed in 1974 (Teasdale & Jennett) the Glasgow Coma Scale (GCS) was a structured approach for assessing levels of consciousness and responsivity in patients with acute brain injury. It has since evolved following feedback from nurses and medical staff and is now an internationally recognized validated tool (Teasdale et al 2014).

The GCS includes assessment of:

+ **Eye** opening
+ **Verbal** response/content of speech
+ **Motor** response/movement of both sides of the body

There are structured ways of stimulating the person to elicit a response if these are not immediately observable and to ensure inter-rater reliability. Also, there are various tools to support its application in practice.

Activity

Access the Glasgow Coma Scale website at *http://www.glasgowcomascale.org/*.

Watch the videos at *http://www.glasgowcomascale.org/#video* and consider the online tools. What is a normal score?

How is the GCS recorded where you work?

Raised intracranial pressure

The pressure within the solid vault of the cranium is influenced by the volume of three components:

+ Brain (e.g. trauma, tumour, abscess)
+ Blood (e.g. aneurysm)
+ Cerebrospinal fluid (CSF) (e.g. meningitis)

An increase or decrease in any component must be met by an alteration in another (Dunn 2002). The body seeks to avoid cerebral ischaemia and subsequent brain damage by maintaining cerebral perfusion. This is achieved by varying cerebral blood flow (cerebral autoregulation) depending on the presence of hypertension or hypotension.

Raised intracranial pressure (ICP) should be suspected if a woman presents with a combination of:

+ Headache
+ Vomiting
+ Altered consciousness
+ Blurred or double vision
+ Photophobia

A doctor would perform a funduscopic examination (using an ophthalmoscope) to look for papilledema, which would indicate raised ICP as CSF bathes the optic nerve. Urgent referral to multi-disciplinary specialists, including neurologists and anaesthetists, will be made to ensure appropriate differential diagnosis, management and care.

Seizures

A seizure happens when the electrical activity of the brain is imbalanced and the cortical brain neurons are temporarily over-excited (Steinert & Froscher 2016). It can cause involuntary body movements which usually last between 30 seconds and 2 minutes, although it can last for longer, and this is called *status epilepticus* (Milligan 2010). Any new seizures or change in mental state should precipitate an urgent neurological assessment (Knight et al 2017).

Women with pre-existing neurological conditions
Epilepsy

Epilepsy is the most common neurological disorder seen in pregnancy, reported to affect about 0.5% to 1% of women of childbearing age (Coad et al 2017), and approximately 2500 women with epilepsy become pregnant (UK and Ireland Epilepsy and Pregnancy Register 2016). It is classified depending on the type of seizure (Table 9.1).

Table 9.1: **Types of seizures**

Partial (limited to a focal area of the brain)	Unimpaired consciousness (simple)
	Impaired consciousness (complex)
Generalized (across both hemispheres of the brain)	Absence 'petit mal'
	Tonic-clonic 'grand mal'
	Atonic (drop attack)
	Myoclonic
	Clonic
	Tonic

Epilepsy can be idiopathic (arising spontaneously with no apparent cause) or secondary and be the result of a brain injury or tumour.

General classifications of epilepsy

Absence seizure

This is a mild form of epilepsy, leading to brief periods of unconsciousness but without convulsions. It starts without warning and lasts a few seconds. The person may appear to be daydreaming and display repetitive movements such as blinking, chewing or tugging at clothes. The seizure ends with the person having no memory that it happened and no after-effects such as confusion. Drug therapy is highly effective but contraindicated in pregnancy. No intervention is required other than informing the person afterwards that they have had an absence seizure and letting them know if they have missed part of the conversation.

Tonic-clonic seizure (grand mal)

During this seizure the person loses consciousness and falls to the floor due to muscle stiffening. They may make a sudden noise due to air passing through the vocal cords and then begin jerking movements. The person may be incontinent, have irregular breathing and appear to froth at the mouth, as they cannot swallow their saliva. The seizure can last a few minutes, but if it lasts more than 5 minutes or they occur in rapid succession, this may be life threatening and require emergency medical intervention. After the event, consciousness is gradually regained, but the person will be drowsy and disorientated for a varying length of time (minutes to days) depending on the individual. This time is known as the *post-ictal state*.

Atonic seizures (drop attacks)

These seizures are characterized by an abrupt loss of consciousness resulting in a fall to the floor. There is no convulsion, and the ability to stand up and walk again returns after a few seconds. This condition may be resistant to drug therapy; therefore precautions against head injury, such as wearing a helmet, may be indicated.

No intervention is required, and the person makes a quick recovery.

Myoclonic seizures

These seizures involve the muscle (myo) and lead to sudden muscle jerking (clonus) in one part of the body, e.g. resulting in a kick, or they can affect the whole body. They are often associated with other types of seizure and can occur in groups (Epilepsy Society 2017). The person remains conscious, and memory is not affected.

> **Activity**
>
> What is Lennox–Gastaut syndrome? When is the peak age of onset, and what types of seizures are associated with this condition?

Clonic seizure

A clonic seizure is associated with jerking movements and potential loss of bodily functions. The person may lose consciousness briefly and be confused afterwards. Over time, the person may go on to develop tonic-clonic seizures.

Tonic seizure

These seizures are rare and can occur throughout the lifespan. They may involve extension or flexion of the limbs or facial and body muscle spasms. They can be grouped with other types of seizures (atonic, absence and myoclonic), in which case they are usually brief and do not involve convulsions. However, when they are prolonged, they become convulsive and are associated with the distressing symptoms seen in the grand mal type of seizure (described earlier).

> **Activity**
>
> Find out what is meant by *pseudoseizures*. What are the clinical features? How are they distinguished from true seizures?

Sudden unexplained death in epilepsy

Women with epilepsy who opt to discontinue anti-epileptic drugs (AEDs) must be fully aware of the risks of status epilepticus and sudden unexplained death in epilepsy (SUDEP) (National Institute for Health and Care Excellence (NICE) 2012, 2018). Such a decision should be discussed and monitored under the care of the epilepsy specialist and contingency measures agreed should the woman's condition deteriorate. In the period covered by a recent confidential enquiry into maternal deaths (Kelso 2017) eight women with epilepsy died: seven in pregnancy, another before her baby was 6 weeks old and another five before their child's first birthday. It was judged that improvements in the management of care could have made a difference to the outcome in 52% of these women. It is therefore vital that midwives know how to provide the most appropriate care to women with epilepsy and are able to offer guidance to enable mothers to take care of their own health.

Management of care

Risk associated with epilepsy

Epilepsy in pregnancy is associated with an increased risk of miscarriage, antepartum and postpartum haemorrhage, reduced fetal growth, induction of labour and caesarean section (Viale et al 2015). Risks to the fetus are associated with the need to intervene for the reasons just noted and also the risks associated with AEDs (see later). Women with epilepsy should receive care coordinated by a team of specialists, including an obstetrician with a special interest, a neurologist and ideally a specialist nurse (Knight et al 2017; Royal College of Obstetricians and Gynaecologists (RCOG) 2016). Only if a woman is seizure-free for 10 years or more and 5 years off AEDs can she be deemed low risk (RCOG 2016).

Pre-conceptual care

In an ideal world, all women should prepare for pregnancy and take stock of their health and lifestyle. However, for women with epilepsy this is particularly important because of their exposure to AEDs. None of the women who died from SUDEP between 2013 and 2015 had their epilepsy under control before they became pregnant (Knight et al 2017:25).

Anti-epileptic drugs

The AED valproate is known to be associated with an increased risk of birth defects: 10 in 100 versus 1 to 2 per 100 in the general population (Medicines & Healthcare Products Regulatory Agency (MHRA) 2018). It should therefore be used with caution in girls and women – only when effective contraception is in place and never in pregnancy (NICE 2012, 2018). Women who conceive on valproate must seek urgent medical review whilst continuing to take their medication. Other AEDs should

Table 9.2: **Relative risk of congenital malformation with AEDs in pregnancy compared with children born to women with untreated epilepsy**

Drug	Relative risk (RR)
Valproate	5.69
Phenytoin	2.38
Carbamazepine	2.01
Lamotrigine	No increased risk
Gabapentin, levetiracetam, oxcarbazepine, primidone, zonisamide	No increased risk, but few studies More research needed

Data from Weston et al (2016).

also be used with caution (Table 9.2) and used under the guidance of a specialist. A pregnancy registry for drug therapy is available to assist in decision-making when considering treatment and fetal safety (Williams & Kehr 2012).

> **Activity**
>
> What other names is valproate known by? What birth defect is it associated with? What contraceptive methods are recommended for women who use valproate?

Folic acid

Folate is a key requirement in the formation of the neural tube of the developing embryo. Pre-conceptual folic acid supplementation is associated with a 62% reduction of the risk of neural tube defects (Blencowe et al 2010) and is recommended for their prevention of (De-Regil et al 2015). NICE (2008, 2017) recommend that all women take 400 micrograms daily for 3 months pre-conceptually and up to 12 weeks of pregnancy. AEDs are known to interfere with folate metabolism; therefore women taking these drugs are recommended to take a higher dose (5 mg/day) during the formation of the neural tube (Shannon et al 2014).

Antenatal care

Whilst it is recommended that women with epilepsy access pre-conceptual care, for those who do not and take themselves off medication, urgent specialist care should be sought to review the most appropriate course of therapeutic action (Knight et al 2017). During a maternal seizure, oxygen supply to the fetus is reduced, and therefore every effort should be made to reduce the frequency and duration of seizures. The importance of adhering to drug regimens must be stressed to the woman and her family, along with the avoidance of stressful or risky activities. Ideally, the pregnancy should be notified to the UK Epilepsy and Pregnancy Register (NICE 2012, 2018) which is collating information about AED use during pregnancy and fetal outcome.

Women should be informed that most women (67%) will not experience a seizure in pregnancy (RCOG 2016).

Labour care

Women with epilepsy should be advised to give birth in a consultant-led unit where one-to-one midwifery support is available, along with facilities for continuous electronic fetal monitoring and neonatal care facilities (RCOG 2016). AEDs should continue throughout labour, and steps should be taken to avoid the triggers for seizures (stress, pain, fatigue, dehydration). Drugs used for the induction of labour are not contraindicated, and the options for analgesia should be carefully considered. Pethidine is not recommended, and birth in water can be offered with caution (RCOG 2016). See Box 9.2 for a summary of actions to be taken if a seizure occurs in labour.

Activity

Consider caring for a woman with epilepsy who wishes to use water in labour. What precautions should be taken to ensure her safety? What is your policy for evacuating a collapsed woman from the pool? What equipment should be close at hand?

Box 9.2 Care during a seizure in labour

- Call for medical assistance.
- Ensure airway is maintained.
- Do not attempt to restrain the person or put something in their mouth.
- Ensure that there is no danger of injury from the immediate environment.
- Establish left lateral tilt and oxygenation.
- Lorazepam given as an intravenous dose of 0.1 mg/kg (usually a 4-mg bolus, with a further dose after 10–20 minutes) is preferred. Diazepam 5–10 mg administered slowly intravenously is an alternative.
- Instigate continuous electronic fetal monitoring.
- After the seizure, maintain position on left side, ensuring a patent airway until she recovers and is gently reassured that she is safe.

From (RCOG 2016)

Postnatal care

After the birth, women with epilepsy should not be cared for in a single room where they cannot be seen (NICE 2012, 2018). However, if they need to stay in hospital in the early postnatal period, it would be optimum if they could be accompanied by a carer, e.g. partner, mother, and this would be best facilitated in a single room whilst ensuring that the woman is not left alone. This constant observation can be difficult for women with epilepsy. Other strategies for women later on in parenthood include changing nappies on the floor and only using very shallow water for baths (Coad et al 2017).

Women with epilepsy are significantly more likely than other mothers to develop depression and anxiety postnatally (Bjørk et al 2015). They and their carers should be alert to the signs and symptoms of deteriorating mental health to enable timely access to appropriate support and treatment.

Contraception

It is important to discuss contraception with women early in the postnatal period so that they can make informed choices about the best option for them. Some hormonal contraceptives are less effective for women taking 'enzyme-inducing' AEDs such as phenytoin and carbamazepine (RCOG 2016). Avoidance of unplanned pregnancy is paramount to ensure appropriate medication and post-birth recovery.

Breastfeeding

Breastfeeding is undoubtedly the most appropriate form of nutrition for babies and is associated with a range of benefits for both the mother and the child in subsequent years (Marshall et al 2017). However, women with epilepsy are particularly vulnerable to the suggestion that they should limit their baby's exposure to AEDs via their breast milk; indeed, the Epilepsy Society leaflet 'Pregnancy and parenting' (2019) advises women to alternate breastfeeds with formula feeds if taking phenobarbital or primidone, as these can make a baby sleepy. However, an extensive review of the literature regarding the benefits and potential harmful effects of exposure of AEDs via breast milk (Velby et al 2015) concluded that most are safe and that some should be used with caution (Table 9.3). In addition, the impact on the baby should be carefully observed and mothers supported practically and emotionally to help them get feeding off to a good start.

With regard to the long-term development of babies exposed to AEDs via breast milk, there is evidence that breastfeeding outweighs any

Table 9.3: **AEDs and breastfeeding**

Safety	AED	Advice
Safe	Phenytoin Valproate Carbamazepine	All babies of mothers taking AEDs should be closely observed for signs of:
Moderate	Lamotrigine Oxcarbazepine Levetiracetam Topiramate Gabapentin Pregabalin Vigabatrin Tiagabine	• Poor suckling • Drowsiness • Jaundice • Rash • Weight gain Mothers should be supported to get adequate rest and hydration
Possibly hazardous	Phenobarbital Primidone Benzodiazepines Clobazam and clonazepam Ethosuximide Zonisamide Felbamate	Mothers should take their AEDs regularly Mothers wishing to stop breastfeeding should do so gradually
No evidence regarding safety (strong caution)	Perampanel Lacosamide Eslicarbazepine	

From (Velby et al 2015)

potential concerns. Indeed, continuous breastfeeding amongst mothers taking AEDs was associated with higher achievement at 6 months compared with babies who did not breastfeed or who stopped early (Velby et al 2013). Women should be informed that there are no known adverse effects in children exposed to AEDs via breast milk (RCOG 2016).

Multiple sclerosis

Multiple sclerosis (MS) is a 'chronic inflammatory demyelinating disease that affects the central nervous system' (Stuart & Bergstrom 2011). The symptoms include:

+ Weakness
+ Numbness of extremities
+ Muscle spasticity
+ Pain
+ Fatigue
+ Bowel and bladder dysfunction
+ Sight changes

Table 9.4: **Categories of multiple sclerosis**

Condition	Description
Relapsing remitting (RRMS)	Most common (85%–90%), characterized by periods of relapse and remission
Secondary progressive (SPMS)	Can develop in people who have had RRMS for some time, leading to exacerbation of symptoms with or without some remissions
Primary progressive (PPMS)	Rare form of MS leading to continued progression and severe impairment of function

Data from Stuart & Bergstrom (2011)

It affects more women than men. The cause is unknown, although environmental and genetic factors are likely to be involved. Interestingly, in a study of 521 patients with MS (Neilsen et al 2016), it was found through examination of their neonatal dried blood spots and comparison with matched controls that low vitamin D levels in the neonate are associated with an increased risk of developing MS – another important reason for encouraging maternal and childhood supplementation as per the Healthy Start Programme (Department of Health 2018).

MS is often categorized depending on the pattern of relapse and remission the person experiences; see Table 9.4.

Pregnancy and MS

A woman planning a pregnancy should seek pre-conceptual counselling specific to her own particular condition and current drug therapy. Some of the treatments for managing MS are teratogenic (e.g. fingolimod), and each has different 'wash-out' periods. It is recommended that women should come off disease-modifying therapies (DMTs) before conception (Lu et al 2012).

The Pregnancy and Multiple Sclerosis (PRIMS) study demonstrated that women have fewer episodes of relapse during pregnancy (Vukusic et al 2004). For women with relapsing MS, the incidence of relapse during pregnancy has been reported at between 17.2% and 13.7% postnatally (Alroughani et al 2018). Relapse rates vary depending on the DMTs used before pregnancy and the length of time they were discontinued for; relapse occurs predominantly in the first and third trimesters.

In women who are in an advanced stage of their disease, pregnancy can pose additional challenges. For example, where there are current bladder problems, pregnant women are more likely to suffer from urinary tract infections (UTIs) and may need antibiotic therapy and to perform additional self-catheterization (Coad et al 2017).

Activity

What is the recommended dose of vitamin D supplementation in pregnancy? Which groups of women should take vitamin D postnatally? What are the risk factors for vitamin D deficiency?

Myasthenia gravis

This autoimmune disease leads to skeletal muscle weakness and fatigue and is caused by interruption of the nerve impulse to the muscle when antibodies block or destroy acetylcholine receptors at the neuromuscular junction. Myasthenia gravis (MG) is more common in women than men and usually presents under the age of 40 years (Grob et al 2008). For some patients, removal of the thymus gland where antibodies are produced provides some improvement of symptoms.

Activity

Access the Myasthenia website at *https://www.myaware.org*. Read some of the case studies to appreciate how the condition first presented and the impact on people's lives.

Pregnancy and childbirth with MG

Some of the drugs used in the management of this condition are known to be teratogenic, e.g. methotrexate, and should not be used within 3 months of a planned pregnancy (Norwood et al 2014). Hence, preconceptual care is advised so that a safe treatment regimen can be established, thus avoiding abrupt removal of therapy or additions of new treatments once a pregnancy is confirmed. A consensus working party came up with a range of recommendations for pregnancy and childbirth care, summarized in Table 9.5.

Up to 30% of infants born to mothers with MG are at risk of developing transient neonatal myasthenia gravis (TNMG) and symptoms of hypotonia and respiratory muscle involvement (Djelmis et al 2002). Hence, intensive neonatal support must be available, including ventilation and possible tube feeding. The condition may have a delayed onset; thus a period of hospital observation of at least 2 days is recommended (Norwood et al 2014).

Table 9.5: **MG best practice care in pregnancy and childbirth**

When	Best practice should include
Pre-conceptual	Consider thymectomy Review of treatment plan and wash-out period for teratogenic drugs
Pregnancy	Multi-professional team care Thyroid function tests Serial scanning for fetal movements monitoring Anaesthetic review
Birth	Consultant-led care Access to onsite intensive care facilities Aim for spontaneous vaginal birth Aim to avoid general anaesthesia where possible IV steroids in labour Avoid magnesium sulphate
Neonatal care	Paediatrician at birth Observation period for TNMG
Postnatal care	Support breastfeeding Neurological review

Data from Norwood et al (2014)

Headache and migraine

Causes of headache are diverse and include:

+ Migraine
+ Pre-eclampsia
+ Tumour
+ Subdural haematoma
+ Subarachnoid haemorrhage
+ Meningitis
+ Stress/non-specific

Migraine affects about 12% of the world's population (Stovner et al 2007) and is two to three times more prevalent in women. It is not surprising therefore that there is a hormonal link, with 50% of women who experience migraine reporting an association with menstruation (Vetvick et al 2014). In a study of 280 women (Petrovski et al 2018), it was reported that women who have menstrual migraine (MM) suffer a higher migraine intensity both in early pregnancy and in the postpartum period than women who do not have MM (nMM). However, the frequency of migraines was lower for both MM and nMM women in the second half of pregnancy and directly after birth.

Headache in pregnancy

Despite the prevalence of migraine, if a woman presents with severe headache in pregnancy or after the birth, consideration must be given to the possibility of pre-eclampsia. In a study of 1101 pregnant women (Melhado et al 2007) of those with no previous history of headache who develop new-onset headache, approximately one-third had pre-eclampsia. The headache associated with pre-eclampsia is usually diffuse, throbbing and constant and may be associated with photophobia and blurred vision. Making a differential diagnosis is important, as blood pressure can also rise due to the associated pain. It is therefore essential that other clinical signs are explored, e.g. epigastric pain, and that biochemical markers such as thrombocytopenia and raised liver enzymes are evaluated (see Chapter 3).

Activity

Review the biochemical markers that are diagnostic for pre-eclampsia. How does the headache associated with migraine differ from that associated with pre-eclampsia?

Postnatal headache

Whilst pre-eclampsia can develop postnatally, another cause of headache after birth is due to post-dural puncture. It is characterized by severe pain, nausea and vomiting when the woman sits upright from the lying position and eased by lying flat again. It is caused by leakage of CSF following puncture of the dura (i.e. after spinal anaesthesia) leading to traction on the intracranial structures. An anaesthetist should be asked to review the woman, and other causes of headache should be excluded.

Activity

Find out the procedure for 'blood patch' where you work. How effective is this method of treatment for post-dural puncture? How should the woman be cared for in these circumstances?

Stroke

Cerebrovascular accident (CVA), or 'stroke', is commonly associated with older age, but younger childbearing women can also experience this life-changing condition. There are two types of stroke:

Table 9.6: **Symptoms of stroke: FAST**

Symptom	Description
Facial weakness	Can the person smile? Does their face droop at one side?
Arm weakness	Can the person raise both arms in the air and keep them there?
Speech problems	Can the person speak clearly and understand what you say?
Time to call 999	If you see any of the three signs, it's time to ring 999.

Adapted from (Stroke Association 2018)

1. Haemorrhagic – bleeding in the brain
2. Ischaemic – blood clot or blockage

A mini-stroke, or transient ischaemic attack (TIA), is described when the symptoms are transient and the blockage is temporary.

Symptoms of stroke

It is important to be able to recognize when a stroke is happening, as prompt treatment can be life-saving. These are summarized in Table 9.6.

Incidence of stroke

In the UK and Ireland between 2013 and 2015 (in pregnancy and up to 6 weeks postnatally):

+ Twelve women died from intracranial haemorrhage
+ Seven women died from subarachnoid haemorrhage
+ Five women died from intracerebral haemorrhage

Another 16 women died from stroke between 6 weeks and 1 year after the end of pregnancy (Knight et al 2017).

As the age of having a baby is increasing, the incidence of stroke in pregnancy is also rising worldwide, impacted by a rise in obesity, hypertension and diabetes (Cauldwell et al 2018).

Treatment of stroke

Women who develop signs of a stroke should receive the same care as the general population: immediate emergency admission and diagnosis via computed tomography (CT) or magnetic resonance imaging (MRI) scan. Treatment will depend on the cause of the stroke: if caused by a bleed, a craniotomy may be required to identify and repair the bleeding point; if caused by a clot, it can be treated with thrombolysis or mechanical thrombectomy (Sheffield Teaching Hospitals 2018). However, one in eight stroke patients will die within 30 days (Stroke Association 2018).

Stroke survivors will require long-term support, including speech and language therapy, physiotherapy, occupational therapy and medication to reduce the risk of further strokes.

Nerve compression

Carpal tunnel syndrome

This distressing condition occurs when the median nerve of the wrist becomes entrapped leading to tingling, pain and numbness in the hand that is generally worse at night. Treatment in pregnancy usually involves wearing a wrist splint, and the condition usually resolves after the birth. Risk factors include increasing maternal age, gestational diabetes and excessive weight gain (Dias et al 2015).

Neurological deficit after birth

On rare occasions women will experience neurological symptoms post-natally. These may be due to the position the woman was in during labour and birth, the position of the fetus, operative delivery or a combination of factors. It is therefore important that those caring for women during birth are mindful of the potential damage to nerves as they support women, especially during prolonged labour and/or spinal anaesthesia. It is important that women are encouraged to change positions frequently and that care is taken not to over-extend leg abduction or prolong thigh flexion.

Women's symptoms will depend on which nerve is involved (Table 9.7). Recovery is usually complete within weeks to 2 years or longer depending on the degree of damage (Howells 2013).

Table 9.7: **Birth-related compression nerve injuries**

Symptom	Cause	Nerves involved
Foot drop; numbness of lateral aspect of thigh, lower leg and dorsum of foot (all on opposite side to position of fetal occiput)	Compression by fetal head during the second stage of labour	L4–L5 S1–S5
Foot drop, numbness of lateral aspect of lower leg and dorsum of foot	Lithotomy/squatting position for prolonged time	L4–L5 S1–S2
Loss of feeling of inner aspect of lower leg and anterior of thigh; difficulty climbing stairs	Compression of femoral nerve during operative birth	L2–L4
Loss of feeling over inner thigh	Compression by fetal head or forceps	L2–L4

Adapted from (Howells 2013) and (Coad et al 2017)

Find out what is meant by the terms *neuropraxia, axonotmesis* and *neurotmesis* in relation to nerve damage. What is the prognosis for each condition?

Ischaemic nerve damage

When the blood supply to a nerve is compromised, damage may occur. Such complications have been reported following the placement of balloon catheters for placenta percreta (Teare et al 2014) and abdominal aorta occlusion during caesarean section (Wei et al 2016).

REFLECTION ON THE TRIGGER SCENARIO

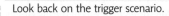

Look back on the trigger scenario.

> Julie and her partner, Joe, are waiting in the hospital antenatal clinic for their detailed scan. Julie was diagnosed with epilepsy when she was 6 years old and has been under the care of a neurologist throughout her childhood. She turns to Joe and says, 'Do you think they will be able to tell if our baby has been damaged by that fit I had last week?'

The scenario is one that illustrates the new journey women with epilepsy embark on. Despite many years of living with the disease women with epilepsy now face the added responsibility of thinking about how their condition might impact on their baby.

Now that you are familiar with the care of pregnant women with epilepsy, you will have insight into how the scenario relates to the evidence. The jigsaw model will now be used to explore the trigger scenario in more depth.

Effective communication

It is paramount that women with epilepsy are given clear and understandable information about what is known about the risks and challenges their condition might pose. This should be communicated pre-conceptually and throughout the pregnancy to ensure that the woman can adjust her behaviour if necessary and not worry unnecessarily. Questions that arise from the scenario include: Did Julie discuss the impact of seizures on fetal wellbeing with her midwife at the booking appointment? What did her midwife inform Julie about the schedule for antenatal care? Who is best placed to discuss the risks and challenges of epilepsy in pregnancy?

Woman-centred care

It is important that women who are managing a chronic condition be involved in decisions about their care. Neurological conditions often develop in a manner that is individual to that person and influenced by a range of environmental and emotional factors, as well as fatigue, general health and how well the disease is managed.

Questions that arise from the scenario might include: Has a personalized care plan been developed for Julie that she was involved in creating? How will Julie's care be managed following her recent seizure? Has Julie reported the seizure to her midwife or care team? How will a woman-centred approach to care be facilitated throughout Julie's pregnancy, birth and postnatal period? Does Julie have access to her own electronic records so she is able to update them?

Using best evidence

The knowledge base about neurological conditions and their impact on childbearing women is growing. It is therefore essential that midwives have access to high-quality, up-to-date evidence to inform their practice and offer choices to women. Such evidence should be regularly synthesized by a multi-professional guideline group that includes key stakeholders, dependent on the guideline under consideration.

Questions that arise from the scenario might include: Did Julie's midwife access the trust guideline on care of a women with epilepsy before she met her? How else might Julie's midwife inform her practice with regard to the latest evidence? What other sources of information can Julie access for herself? What reputable sources can midwives direct women to?

Professional and legal issues

Midwives must always ensure that they provide care within the professional and legal framework that supports effective care. They must ensure that all procedures offered to women are preceded by relevant information that enables them to make an informed decision. Questions that arise from the scenario might include: Has Julie been informed what the detailed scan is for and what it can and cannot identify? When written consent is not required for a procedure, how should the decision-making process be documented? How long are maternity records required to be kept?

Caring for women with complex medical conditions requires close and coordinated care by the multi-professional team. During pregnancy the midwife is key to ensuring that the woman is able to follow the pro-gramme of care required and that she has sufficient information and support to adhere to it. Questions that arise from the scenario might include: Who is the lead professional for Julie throughout her preg-nancy? What plans are in place to enable Julie to have timely access to her neurologist if needed? How will the maternity care record facilitate effective team working? Who will Julie see after her scan? Which addi-tional professionals will be involved in Julie's maternity care?

Developing and maintaining clinical midwifery skills is fundamental to ensuring that women have confidence in their midwife. Being able to use monitoring equipment, take blood and perform an abdominal examination all contribute to her perception that she is in safe hands. Questions that arise from the scenario might include: What has Julie's experience been of neurological care before she became pregnant? What are her expectations in relation to receiving skilled and effect-ive care from her maternity care team? What additional tests will the midwife need to perform during Julie's pregnancy journey?

Current UK maternity policy *Better Births* (National Maternity Review 2016) requires maternity services to develop continuity pathways for most women. Continuity of carer is known to lead to less interven-tion and better outcomes for women and their babies (Sandall et al 2013). Women with complex conditions such as epilepsy who expe-rience a continuity of carer model where their care is provided by a lead midwife working in a team of four to eight other midwives are more likely to experience seamless, coordinated care. Questions that arise from the scenario might include: How will Julie continue to see her lead community midwife if she is having consultant-led care? How will Julie meet all members of the team? How can Julie receive care in labour by a midwife she has already met?

Ensuring a safe environment is paramount for women with epilepsy, and no more so when they become pregnant and anticipate the birth of their baby. Women with epilepsy can be reluctant to keep taking their medication due to fears that it will harm their baby. They will also need to plan for parenting in an environment that ensures they minimize the potential risk of having a seizure while holding the baby or bathing, etc. Having a known midwife throughout pregnancy will also enhance safety, as a personalized care plan can be developed with the woman and reviewed at each antenatal visit. Questions that arise from the scenario might include: Did Julie have pre-conceptual care and a medication review before she became pregnant? Was her recent seizure because she has changed or reduced her medication? At what point in pregnancy should discussions start about preparing for the baby at home? How can the midwife support Julie to create a safe home for her baby?

Promotes health

Pregnancy is an opportunity for health professionals to offer support for women to adopt healthy habits and address any potentially harmful behaviours, such as smoking or a sedentary lifestyle. Making every antenatal and postnatal contact count is optimum but should be carefully undertaken to avoid the person feeling judged. Questions that arise from the scenario might include: What opportunities might arise during a detailed scan for lifestyle issues to be raised? How should public health messages be conveyed? What methods are used where you work for getting information across to women in a non-judgemental way? How can opportunities be maximized to involve partners and parents in any discussions which promote healthy options?

Further scenarios

The following scenarios enable you to consider how specific situations influence the care the midwife provides. Use the jigsaw model to explore the issues raised in the scenario.

SCENARIO 1

Alison has gone back to bed with a terrible headache. She is 30 weeks pregnant and feels too ill to go to work. Matt, her partner, is worried about her, and when she doesn't answer his text, he decides to pop back home at lunch time to see how Alison is. He goes into the bedroom and when he calls her name, assumes she has fallen asleep. However, when he goes over to Alison, he notices that the side of her mouth is drooping, and her arm is hanging awkwardly over the side of the bed. He tries to rouse her, and she half-opens her eyes and tries to talk but does not make any sense.

Stroke is a life-threatening event that may be caused by a bleed or a clot on the brain. This can lead to ischaemia and brain damage if not treated quickly and effectively. There have been numerous public health campaigns alerting members of the public how to recognize the signs and not delay in seeking urgent attention.

Questions that could be asked are:

1. What action should Matt take?
2. If Matt chose to ring the maternity unit for advice, what should the midwife recommend?
3. What are the likely causes of a stroke in a woman of childbearing age?
4. What factors increase the risk of a pregnant women having a stroke?
5. What are the chances of Alison making a full recovery?
6. What support services will she need throughout her rehabilitation?

SCENARIO 2

Katie is 16 years of age and has epilepsy. She has been taking valproate for the last 5 years, and it has been the most effective treatment she has used. Katie is surprised, however, at the next neurology appointment when the nurse asks her about contraception. Her mother, who is with her, says, 'Oh she doesn't need to worry about that, do you, darling?' Katie looks sheepish and blushes.

Increasing evidence about the teratogenic effect of valproate has led to a targeted campaign to raise awareness in young women with epilepsy and for the health professionals who care for them. It is known that this drug, whilst an effective treatment for epilepsy, can lead to birth defects and learning and learning problems in children born to mothers who take this drug in pregnancy.

Questions that could be asked are:

1. What other names is valproate known by?
2. What birth defects is valproate associated with?
3. What methods of contraception might be the best option for Katie?
4. How can health professionals avoid the embarrassing situation described here?

5. How long should women be off valproate before they try for a baby?
6. What options should be available to women who conceive while taking valproate?

Conclusion

There are many neurological conditions that women may already have before they become pregnant. Such women will need careful counselling about how these might be affected by pregnancy and childbirth. Women are also at risk of developing a neurological condition or insult during their childbearing journey, and it is important that a full and comprehensive examination is undertaken on women who present with any potential signs or symptoms suggestive of neurological deficit. Specialist input is imperative, and maintaining continuity of midwifery care is the gold standard.

Resources

MS Society https://www.mssociety.org.uk

UK epilepsy in pregnancy register http://www.epilepsyandpregnancy.co.uk

Valproate information resources. Medicines & Healthcare products Regulatory Agency https://www.gov.uk/drug-safety-update/valproate-medicines-epilim-depakote-pregnancy-prevention-programme-materials-online?utm_source=eshot&utm_medium=email&utm_campaign=DSUMay2018Split1

Glasgow coma score observation chart https://www.gla.ac.uk/media/media_19594_en.pdf

Myasthenia Gravis support. Myaware https://www.myaware.org/myasthenia-gravis

Stroke Association https://www.stroke.org.uk/

References

Alroughani, R., Alowayesh, M., Ahmed, S., et al., 2018. Relapse occurrence in women with multiple sclerosis during pregnancy in the new treatment era. Neurology 90 (10), E840–E846.

Bjørk, M., Veiby, G., Reiter, S., et al., 2015. Depression and anxiety in women with epilepsy during pregnancy and after delivery: a prospective population-based cohort study on frequency, risk factors, medication and prognosis. Epilepsia 56 (1), 28–39. doi:10.1111/epi.12884.

Blencowe, H., Cousens, S., Modell, B., Lawn, J., 2010. Folic acid to reduce neonatal mortality from neural tube disorders. Int. J. Epidemiol. 39, i110–i121.

Cauldwell, M., Rudd, A., Nelson-Piercy, C., 2018. Management of stroke and pregnancy. Eur. Stroke J. 3 (3), 227–236.

Coad, F., Mohan, A., Nelson-Piercy, C., 2017. Neurological disease in pregnancy. Obstet. Gynaecol. Reprod. Med. 27 (5), 137–143. Web.

Department of Health (2018) Healthy Start Programme https://www.healthystart.nhs.uk/.

De-Regil, L., Peña-Rosas, J., Fernández-Gaxiola, A.C., Rayco-Solon, P., 2015. Effects and safety of periconceptional oral folate supplementation for preventing birth defects. Cochrane Database Syst. Rev. (12), Art. No.: CD007950, doi:10.1002/14651858.CD007950.pub3.

Dias, G., Santini, A., Vianna, L., et al., 2015. Risk factors of carpal tunnel syndrome in pregnancy. Int. J. Epidemiol. 44, 88.

Djelmis, J., Sostarko, M., Mayer, D., et al., 2002. Myasthenia gravis in pregnancy: report on 69 cases. Eur. J. Obstet. Gynecol. Reprod. Biol. 104, 21–25.

Dunn, L., 2002. Raised intracranial pressure. J. Neurol. Neurosurg. Psychiatry 73 (Suppl. 1), I23–I27.

Epilepsy Society, 2017. https://www.epilepsysociety.org.uk.

Epilepsy Society, 2019. Pregnancy and parenting. https://www.epilepsysociety. org.uk/system/files/attachments/PregnancyandparentingApril2019_11.pdf.

Grob, D., Brunner, N., Namba, T., et al., 2008. Lifetime course of myasthenia gravis. Muscle Nerve 37, 141–149.

Howells, A., 2013. Neurological complications in obstetric regional anaesthesia. Anaesth. Intensive Care Med. 14 (8), 331–332.

Kelso, A., Wills, A., Knight, M., on behalf of the MBRRACE-UK neurology chapter writing group, 2017. Lessons on epilepsy and stroke. In: Knight, M., Nair, M., Tuffnell, D., et al. on behalf of MBRRACE-UK (Eds.), Saving Lives, Improving Mothers' Care – Lessons Learned to Inform Maternity Care From the UK and Ireland Confidential Enquiries Into Maternal Deaths and Morbidity 2013–15. National Perinatal Epidemiology Unit, University of Oxford, Oxford, pp. 24–36.

Knight, M., Kenyon, S., Brocklehurst, P., et al. on behalf of MBRRACE-UK (Eds.), 2014. Saving Lives, Improving Mothers' Care – Lessons learned to inform future maternity care from the UK and Ireland Confidential Enquiries into Maternal Deaths and Morbidity 2009–12. Oxford: National Perinatal Epidemiology Unit, University of Oxford.

Knight, M., Tuffnell, D., Kenyon, S., et al. on behalf of MBRRACE-UK (Eds.), 2015. Saving Lives, Improving Mothers' Care – Surveillance of maternal deaths in the UK 2011–13 and lessons learned to inform maternity care from the UK and Ireland Confidential Enquiries into Maternal Deaths and Morbidity 2009–13. Oxford: National Perinatal Epidemiology Unit, University of Oxford.

Knight, M., Nair, M., Tuffnell, D., et al. on behalf of MBRRACE-UK, 2017. Saving Lives, Improving Mothers' Care – Lessons Learned to Inform Maternity Care From the UK and Ireland Confidential Enquiries Into Maternal Deaths and Morbidity 2013–15. National Perinatal Epidemiology Unit, University of Oxford, Oxford.

Lu, E.W., Wang, B., Guimond, C., et al., 2012. Disease-modifying drugs for multiple sclerosis in pregnancy: a systematic review. Neurology 79 (11), 1130–1135.

Marshall, J., Baston, H., Hall, J., 2017. Midwifery Essentials, vol. 5. Infant Feeding Elsevier, Edinburgh.

Medicines and Healthcare products Regulatory Agency (MHRA), 2018. https:// www.gov.uk/drug-safety-update/valproate-medicines-epilim-depakote-pregnancy-prevention-programme-materials-online.

Melhado, E., Maciel, J., Guerreiro, C., 2007. Headache during gestation: evaluation of 1101 women. Can. J. Neurol. Sci. 34 (2), 187.

Milligan, T., 2010. Status epilepticus. In: Mushlin, S., Greene, H. (Eds.), Decision Making in Medicine. An Algorithmic Approach, 3rd ed. Mosby, Philadelphia.

National Institute for Health and Care Excellence (NICE) 2008, updated 2017 Antenatal care: for uncomplicated pregnancies. CG62. https://www.nice.org.uk/guidance/cg62.

National Institute for Health and Care Excellence (NICE 2012, updated 2018) National Institute for Health and Care Excellence Epilepsies: diagnosis and management. https://www.nice.org.uk/guidance/cg137.

National Maternity Review (2016) Better Births. Improving outcomes of maternity services in England. Available at: https://www.england.nhs.uk/wp-content/uploads/2016/02/national-maternity-review-report.pdf.

Nielsen, N., Munger, K., Koch-Henriksen, N., et al., 2016. Neonatal vitamin D status and risk of multiple sclerosis: a population-based case-control study. Neurology 88 (1), doi:10.1212/WNL.0000000000003454.

Norwood, F., Dhanjal, M., Hill, M., et al., 2014. Myasthenia in pregnancy: best practice guidelines from a UK multispecialty working group. J. Neurol. Neurosurg. Psychiatry 85 (5), 538–543.

Petrovski, B., Vetvik, K., Lundqvist, K., Eberhard-Gran, G., 2018. Characteristics of menstrual versus non-menstrual migraine during pregnancy: a longitudinal population-based study. J. Headache Pain 19 (1), 1–9.

Royal College of Obstetricians and Gynaecologists 2016. Epilepsy in pregnancy. Green Top Guideline No. 68 https://www.rcog.org.uk/globalassets/documents/guidelines/green-top-guidelines/gtg68_epilepsy.pdf.

Sandall, J., Gates, S., Shennan, A., Devane, D., 2013. Midwife-led continuity models versus other models of care for childbearing women. Cochrane Database Syst. Rev. (8), CD004667.

Shannon, G., Alberg, C., Nacul, L., Pashayan, N., 2014. Preconception healthcare and congenital disorders: systematic review of the effectiveness of preconception care programs in the prevention of congenital disorders. Matern. Child Health J. 18 (6), 1354–1379.

Sheffield Teaching Hospitals NHS Foundation Trust (2018). Woman who suffered stroke at 39 weeks pregnant saved by procedure to mechanically remove clot from brain. https://www.sth.nhs.uk/news/news?action=view&newsID=1067.

Steinert, T., Froscher, W., 2016. Major neurological and neuromuscular adverse effects of antipsychotic drugs. In: Manu, P., Flanagan, R., Ronaldson, K. (Eds.), Life-Threatening Effects of Antipsychotic Drugs. Elsevier.

Stovner, L., Hagen, K., Jensen, R., et al., 2007. The global burden of headache: a documentation of headache prevalence and disability worldwide. Cephalalgia 27 (3), 193–210.

Stroke Association (2018) https://www.stroke.org.uk/what-is-stroke/types-of-stroke.

Stuart, M., Bergstrom, L., 2011. Pregnancy and multiple sclerosis. J. Midwifery Womens Health 56 (1), 41–47.

Teasdale, G., Jennett, B., 1974. Assessment of coma and impaired consciousness. Lancet 2, 81–84.

Teasdale, G., Maas, A., Lecky, F., et al., 2014. The glasgow coma scale at 40 years: standing the test of time. Lancet Neurol. 13 (8), 844–854.

Teare, J., Evans, E., Belli, A., Wendler, R., 2014. Sciatic nerve ischaemia after iliac artery occlusion balloon catheter placement for placenta percreta. Int. J. Obstet. Anesth. 23 (2), 178–181.

UK and Ireland Epilepsy Register, 2016. http://www.epilepsyandpregnancy.co.uk.

Veiby, G., Bjørk, M., Engelsen, B., Gilhus, N., 2015. Epilepsy and recommendations for breastfeeding. Seizure 28 (C), 57–65.

Veiby, G., Engelsen, B., Gilhus, N., 2013. Early child development and exposure to antiepileptic drugs prenatally and through breastfeeding: a prospective cohort study on children of women with epilepsy. JAMA Neurol. 70, 1367–1374.

Vetvik, K., Macgregor, A., Lundqvist, C., Russell, M., 2014. Prevalence of menstrual migraine: a population-based study. Cephalalgia 34 (4), 280–288.

Viale, L., Allotey, J., Cheong-See, F., et al., 2015. Epilepsy in pregnancy and reproductive outcomes: a systematic review and meta-analysis. Lancet 386 (10006), 1845–1852.

Vukusic, S., Hutchinson, M., Hours, M., et al., 2004. Pregnancy and multiple sclerosis (the PRIMS study): Clinical predictors of postpartum relapse. Brain 127 (6), 1353–1360.

Wei, X., Zhang, J., Chu, Q., et al., 2016. Prophylactic abdominal aorta balloon occlusion during caesarean section: a retrospective case series. Int. J. Obstet. Anesth. 27 (C), 3–8.

Weston, J., Bromley, R., Jackson, C., et al., 2016. Monotherapy treatment of epilepsy in pregnancy: congenital malformation outcomes in the child. Cochrane Database Syst. Rev. (11), Art. No.: CD010224, doi:10.1002/14651858. CD010224.pub2.

Williams, S., Kehr, H., 2012. An Update in the Treatment of Neurologic Disorders During Pregnancy—Focus on Migraines and Seizures. J. Pharm. Pract. 25 (3), 341–351.

CHAPTER 10

Endocrine disorders and pregnancy

TRIGGER SCENARIO

Rebecca was diagnosed with type 1 diabetes when she was 8 years old. She and her parents have always managed her diabetes carefully, following the diet, exercise and insulin therapy advised by her diabetes team. She is now 26 years old and in a stable relationship with Matt. They are hoping to start a family soon but are aware that there is an increased chance of complications for pregnant women with diabetes and their babies. Matt plans to attend Rebecca's next appointment with the diabetic team so that they can discuss how to avoid or minimize these potential complications.

Introduction

The endocrine system is involved in the regulation of all bodily functions and has the potential to cause a wide range of disorders when its ability to maintain homeostasis is impaired. This chapter provides an overview of the endocrine system and outlines some of the endocrine disorders that affect women's ability to conceive, their pregnancy experiences and the outcomes for themselves and their babies. Midwives are likely to encounter some of these disorders, such as gestational diabetes, more frequently than others. Having some understanding of the less commonly encountered endocrine disorders in pregnancy, such as pituitary or adrenal adenomas, is a useful addition to the midwife's background knowledge.

Physiology

The endocrine system works in conjunction with the nervous system to control bodily functions. Actions of the two systems (neuroendocrine) are linked by the hypothalamus, which controls endocrine gland functioning through negative and positive feedback systems. Endocrine glands contain secretory cells which produce and release hormones into the bloodstream to be carried to specific target tissues. Some hormones are released directly into extracellular fluid to act on local tissue; paracrine hormones act on different types of tissue, and autocrine hormones act on the same kind of tissue. Hormones are concerned with precise regulation and can take anything from seconds to days to take effect (Matthews & Rankin 2017). Endocrine glands include the pituitary, thyroid, parathyroid, adrenal and pineal gland. The pituitary gland has two lobes: anterior and posterior. The anterior gland (master endocrine gland) produces and releases hormones; the posterior gland stores and releases hypothalamic hormones (Matthews & Rankin 2017). Table 10.1 provides an overview of the pituitary hormones and their actions.

The organs which are also involved in the secretion of hormones include the pancreas, ovaries, testes and placenta (Matthews & Rankin 2017). The pancreas contains groups of cells (islets of Langerhans)

Table 10.1: Pituitary hormones and their actions

Anterior pituitary hormones	Action
Thyroid-stimulating hormone (TSH)	Stimulates growth and activity of thyroid gland Release of thyroid hormones under negative feedback system • Thyroxine (T_4) • Tri-iodothyronine (T_3) Thyroid hormones regulate metabolism
Adrenocorticotrophic hormone (ACTH)	Acts on the adrenal cortex, which produces three groups of hormones: • Mineralocorticoids – regulate water and electrolyte balance • Glucocorticoids (steroids), including cortisol (hydrocortisone) – regulate metabolism and response to stress • Sex hormones (gonadocorticoids)
Follicle-stimulating hormone (FSH)	Involved in control of menstrual cycle
Luteinizing hormone (LH)	Involved in control of menstrual cycle
Growth hormone	Stimulates growth and division of cells (highest levels produced during sleep)
Prolactin	Stimulates production of breast milk
Posterior pituitary hormones	Action
Oxytocin	Stimulates myometrial contraction Stimulates ejection of breast milk
Anti-diuretic hormone (ADH)	Inhibits production of urine and increases blood volume

which produce glucagon (α cells) and insulin (β cells) to control blood sugar levels and the metabolism of fat, protein and glucose (Matthews & Rankin 2017).

What are your pre-conceptions about why someone might have diabetes? Do you know anyone with diabetes? What do you know about the long-term consequences of this condition? How might these be avoided?

Diabetes

'Diabetes mellitus is characterised by impaired carbohydrate utilisation caused by an absolute or relative deficiency of insulin production by the endocrine pancreas' (Rankin 2017:361). Inadequate levels of insulin mean inadequate levels of glucose are available to the tissues. The body responds by attempting to provide energy through gluconeogenesis and the release of protein and fats (Fig. 10.1). This results in hyperglycaemia, glycosuria, polyuria, dehydration and increased thirst, ketonuria, metabolic acidosis and lowered blood pH levels. If uncorrected, acidosis can lead to coma and death (Rankin 2017). Diabetes has widespread

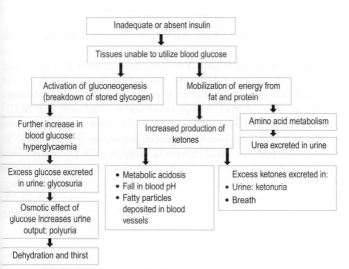

Fig. 10.1 Physiological impact of inadequate insulin production. (Developed from Rankin 2017.)

effects; it is also associated with higher mortality from cardiovascular and renal diseases, retinopathy and possible blindness, hypertension and stroke. Infections thrive on the excess glucose available, and blood vessels become damaged. There are different types of diabetes, which will be summarized next.

Type 1 diabetes

With type 1 diabetes, there is almost no production of insulin. Therefore, people with this type require insulin treatment: insulin-dependent diabetes (IDDM). IDDM is subdivided into two types:

+ IDDM type 1A: develops in childhood; is associated with genetic and environmental factors
+ IDDM type 1B: develops in adulthood; is probably genetic (Rankin 2017)

Type 2 diabetes

Non-insulin-dependent diabetes mellitus (NIDDM) is more common than IDDM. It is associated with obesity, older maternal age and some ethnic origins and is more common in areas of social deprivation (Health Quality Improvement Partnership (HQIP) 2017). Insulin is less able to facilitate cellular uptake of glucose; there is insulin resistance (Rankin 2017).

Gestational diabetes mellitus

Gestational diabetes mellitus (GDM) is when diabetes first arises during pregnancy. The production of insulin is inadequate to meet the woman's needs during pregnancy and may reflect chronic β-cell dysfunction: diabetes-in-waiting. Detecting dysfunction through blood glucose screening can identify women for whom the development of diabetes can be averted or delayed through interventions (Buchanan et al 2007). The rate of GDM has increased recently and is considered to reflect the incidence of type 2 diabetes in the general population (Ferrara 2007). It is associated with hormonal changes in pregnancy (in particular, corticosteroids and progesterone), familial tendencies and impaired glucose response to stress (Rankin 2017). Women who are obese and develop GDM may be especially likely to develop type 2 diabetes later in life (Rankin 2017), and around 50% of women with GDM can develop type 2 diabetes within 5 years of the affected pregnancy (Ferrara 2007).

Diabetes and pregnancy

The National Pregnancy in Diabetes Audit 2016 (HQIP 2017) reported on the pregnancies of 3297 women with diabetes in England, Wales and the Isle of Man. Almost half of these women had type 2 diabetes, and of those almost half were of Black, Asian or mixed ethnic origin. Diabetes can be more difficult to control during pregnancy, although pregnant women with impaired glucose tolerance may not show signs of the disease (Rankin 2017) (see Table 10.2 for an overview of the blood tests relating to diabetes). As pregnancy advances, insulin resistance increases under the influence of placental hormones, and greater amounts of insulin are required. In 2016, almost 10% of pregnant women with type 1 diabetes were admitted to hospital with severe hypoglycaemia, and 2.7% of this group of women were admitted to hospital at least once with diabetic ketoacidosis (HQIP 2017). Specific complications are associated with diabetes during pregnancy. These include diabetic retinopathy, diabetic nephropathy, hypertensive disorders, congenital anomalies and issues with fetal growth.

Diabetic retinopathy

Diabetic retinopathy affects women's vision and is associated with poor glycaemic control, hypertension, proteinuria and poor perinatal outcomes.

Table 10.2: **Blood testing in diabetes**

The test	Information
HBA1c (glycated haemoglobin)	Measures the excess blood glucose attached to red blood cells
	Assesses the average blood glucose over previous 2–3 months, using a sample of blood
	Raised levels indicate a higher risk of developing complications of diabetes
	Factors that can affect readings include:
	• Illness
	• Medication, e.g. steroids
	• Lifestyle changes
	• Stress or depression
	Target levels differ according to type of diabetes (e.g. type 1 diabetics: <48 mmol/L; people at risk of diabetes: 42–47 mmol/L) (Diabetes UK 2018)
	Women whose HBA1c is >86 mmol/L: advised to avoid pregnancy due to risk of complications (NICE 2015)
	Measuring HBA1c during pregnancy:
	• At booking and during second and third trimesters for women with pre-existing diabetes (increased risk linked with HBA1c >48 mmol/L)
	• At diagnosis of GDM to identify type 2 diabetes (NICE 2015)

Continued

Table 10.2: **Blood testing in diabetes** *(Continued)*

The test	Information
Capillary blood glucose test (finger prick)	Self-blood glucose monitoring for people with diabetes Target capillary glucose levels for type 1 diabetes (pre-conception) • 5–7 mmol/L on waking • 4–7 mmol/L pre-meals at other times Daily recommendations for testing during pregnancy: women with type 1 diabetes or who are on multiple-dose insulin therapy • Fasting • Pre-meal • 1 hour post-meal • Bedtime Daily recommendations for testing during pregnancy: women on diet and exercise therapy, oral therapy or once-daily insulin • Fasting • 1 hour post-meal Target capillary glucose levels during pregnancy • Fasting: ≤5.3 mmol/L • 1 hour post-meal ≤7.8 mmol/L • 2 hours post-meal ≤6.4 mmol/L To avoid hypoglycaemia capillary glucose levels should be ≥4 mmol/L (NICE 2015)
Oral glucose tolerance test (OGTT)	2-hour 75-g OGTT – recommended screening test for GDM Offered at 24–28 weeks' gestation for women with one or more risk factors for GDM Offered in early pregnancy for women with GDM in a previous pregnancy; if early OGTT is normal, it is repeated at 28 weeks GDM is diagnosed if: • Fasting blood glucose ≥5.6 mmol/L OR • 2-hour blood glucose ≥7.8 mmol/L (NICE 2015)
Fasting blood glucose	Not recommended as a screening test for GDM due to low sensitivity (Whitelaw & Gayle 2010)
Blood ketone (ketonaemia) testing	Home blood ketone testing can be performed by women with type 1 diabetes in case of hyperglycaemia or feeling unwell Women with type 2 diabetes or GDM should seek medical advice urgently if they become hyperglycaemic or feel unwell Women with any form of diabetes who are hyperglycaemic or unwell should have urgent testing for ketonaemia to exclude ketoacidosis (NICE 2015)

Excellent control of blood glucose levels and blood pressure with frequent retinal examinations are an important aspect of pre-conceptual and antenatal care (Rankin 2017). Where women have diabetic retinopathy, postnatal follow-up care from an ophthalmologist is recommended for at least 6 months (National Institute for Health and Care Excellence (NICE) 2015).

Diabetic nephropathy

Diabetic nephropathy is also known as *diabetic kidney disease*; it affects some people with diabetes causing excessive proteinuria, lesions in the renal glomeruli and diminished glomerular filtration rate. Diabetic nephropathy affects people to varying degrees but can ultimately lead to end-stage renal disease (Lim 2014). In pregnancy it is linked with pre-eclampsia, prematurity and growth restriction for the baby (Kourtis 2012). Careful monitoring is linked with good outcomes (Rankin 2017), and involvement of a nephrologist is important if renal function is impaired. Nephrotic-range proteinuria (>5 g/day) is associated with an increased risk of venous thromboembolism (VTE), and VTE prophylaxis may be indicated (NICE 2015).

Hypertension

Hypertensive disorders are more likely in women with diabetes who have pre-existing vascular problems. They are more likely to develop pre-eclampsia, fetal growth restriction and placental abruption (Starikov et al 2015). Anti-platelet agents such as aspirin may be offered to reduce the risk of pre-eclampsia. Some anti-hypertensive drugs can be potentially harmful during pregnancy. Therefore, women with pre-existing diabetes who are also hypertensive may need their anti-hypertensive treatment replaced with alternative drugs beginning in the pre-conception period (HQIP 2017). For further information about hypertensive disorders in pregnancy, see Chapter 3.

Fetal, neonatal and childhood issues

Pregnancy complicated by pre-existing diabetes and gestational diabetes can affect fetal, neonatal and childhood short- and long-term health. Maternal hyperglycaemia leads to increased fetal hyperglycaemia and increased insulin levels, resulting in an accumulation of fat and disproportionate growth. Increased growth requires additional oxygenation which, if unmet, can lead to placental and fetal hypoxia. Hypoglycaemia is also associated with adverse fetal adverse outcomes (Starikov et al 2015).

Improved screening, treatment and monitoring of maternal diabetes have reduced the incidence of associated stillbirths in recent years. However, in comparison to the wider population, HQIP (2017) reported twice as many stillbirths and four times as many neonatal deaths in women with diabetes. A significant number of stillbirths have been linked with missed opportunities to identify and offer testing to women at risk for diabetes, as well as monitoring fetal growth (Manktelow et al 2017). In addition, congenital anomalies occurred more frequently in mothers with both type 1 (47.6 per 1000) and type 2 (44.8 per 1000) diabetes (HQIP 2017). Congenital anomalies include fetal cardiomyopathy and cardiovascular anomalies, neural tube defects, musculoskeletal defects and gastrointestinal defects (Starikov et al 2015). Adverse fetal outcomes are particularly associated with high maternal HBA_{1c} levels during the pre-conceptual and early pregnancy periods. However, over 90% of women with diabetes could be better prepared for pregnancy, and women from the most deprived groups are the least prepared (HQIP 2017).

Babies of mothers with diabetes also have a higher risk of being born preterm or sustaining birth trauma as a consequence of events such as shoulder dystocia, particularly if maternal HBA_{1c} is greater than 8.5% (Starikov et al 2015) and the fetus is macrosomic (birth weight ≥4 kg). Longer-term risks for the infant include higher incidence of childhood obesity and type 2 diabetes in adulthood. These children may have a shorter attention span and more problems with language (Whitelaw & Gayle 2011).

Antenatal care

The aims of diabetic management during pregnancy are to maintain normal maternal blood glucose levels through:

+ Monitoring blood glucose levels regularly and frequently
+ Maintaining a controlled diet
+ Anti-diabetic (hypoglycaemic) medical management (for instance, metformin, insulin or both)

For an overview of recommended lifestyle and medical interventions for women with diabetes in pregnancy, see Table 10.3. There is variation between countries in strategies for detecting GDM, although at least one of the following strategies is generally adopted: assessment of clinical risk and glucose tolerance testing. The booking appointment is an ideal opportunity for midwives to identify women who are more likely to develop GDM based on recognized risk factors:

+ Body mass index (BMI) >30 kg/m^2
+ Previous baby weighing ≥4.5 kg
+ Previous GDM

Table 10.3: **Management of diabetes in pregnancy**

Intervention	
Diet	Ethnically appropriate dietary advice from dietician/ nutritionist, including: • Restricted carbohydrates, with a preference for carbohydrates with low-glycaemic index, e.g. whole grain foods • High-fibre foods, e.g. vegetables • Portion control
Activity	Increased activity helps control diabetes In pregnancy, this can include swimming, walking and yoga (Whitelaw & Gayle 2010)
Blood glucose monitoring	To monitor condition and regulate therapy
Medical management	Required in 10%–20% women with GDM (Murphy 2010)
Insulin	Aids in tight control of blood glucose levels Offered when: • Usual management is with insulin • Diet and activity fail to control blood glucose levels in GDM • Fasting blood glucose ≥7.0 mmol/L at diagnosis of GDM • Fasting blood glucose 6.0–6.9 mmol/L with complications, e.g. macrosomia, polyhydramnios • If oral hypoglycaemics are contraindicated (NICE 2015) Types: • Short acting • Long acting
Oral hypoglycaemics	Metformin • Increases insulin sensitivity • Considered safe in all trimesters (Whitelaw & Gayle 2010), although it does cross the placenta • Not associated with maternal hypoglycaemia (Murphy 2010) • Only oral hypoglycaemic drug recommended in pre-conception period and pregnancy (NICE 2015) Glibenclamide • Enhances insulin secretion • Minimal transfer across the placenta (Whitelaw & Gayle 2010) • Considered if metformin is not tolerated • Considered if metformin does not achieve target blood glucose levels and insulin is declined (NICE 2015)

+   First-degree relative with diabetes
+   Family ethnic origin has a high prevalence of diabetes

Women who present with one or more of these factors should be offered testing for GDM using a 75-g glucose tolerance test in accordance with the findings of the multi-national Hyperglycemia and Adverse Pregnancy Outcome (HAPO) study (International Association of Diabetes and Pregnancy Study Groups Consensus 2010) so that appropriate management can be provided if GDM is diagnosed.

Positive results from glucose tolerance testing identify a small number of women who would be diabetic outside pregnancy, and higher numbers of women are at increased risk of developing type 2 diabetes at a later date (Buchanan et al 2007). The RADIEL study (Koivusalo et al 2016) found that individualized modest lifestyle changes such as dietary modifications and increased physical activity could reduce the risk of GDM by 39% for women who are at high risk for developing this condition. Effective management of GDM can be beneficial in terms of maternal weight, birth weight of the baby, pre-eclampsia and gestational hypertension and mode of birth and, for women with moderate GDM, can reduce the likelihood of severe perinatal problems (Murphy 2010).

Management of diabetes includes providing the woman with information about diabetes in pregnancy and making a referral to the multi-disciplinary antenatal diabetes team before 10 weeks' gestation or within 1 week of diagnosis for GDM (NICE 2015). Offering women with diabetes a higher dose of folic acid (5 mg daily) can reduce the increased risk of neural tube defects (HQIP 2017). Congenital anomalies can be detected during the routinely offered 20-week ultrasound scan (NICE 2015) or fetal echocardiogram. Additional serial (monthly) ultrasound scans to monitor fetal growth and liquor volume are offered from 28 to 36 weeks' gestation and, where there are concerns about fetal or maternal health, assessment of fetal wellbeing should be arranged accordingly. This can include electronic fetal monitoring, biophysical profiling, amniotic fluid indexing and fetal umbilical Doppler recordings (NICE 2015). Identification of macrosomia is also important, although ultrasound measurements can be inaccurate by 15% (Starikov et al 2015).

Activity

Access the NICE (2015) guidelines for managing diabetes in pregnancy. Look at the schedule for antenatal appointments and compare these with the guidelines in your placement area. Are there any differences in the two sets of guidance? Arrange to spend time in a joint antenatal diabetes clinic to get a better understanding of women's experiences.

Labour and birth

Maternal diabetes is associated with higher rates of preterm birth, particularly for women with type 1 diabetes (43.3%) (HQIP 2017). If preterm birth is likely and maternal antenatal steroids are indicated for maturing the fetal lungs, this can increase maternal blood glucose levels. Where the mother's blood glucose levels are being managed with insulin, the dose should be increased accordingly. In preparation for labour and birth, women should have an opportunity for discussions about the timing and mode of birth with the specialist team, particularly in the third trimester. Consideration is given to the type of diabetes and the presence of any maternal or fetal complications, such as macrosomia (NICE 2015). Women with type 1 and type 2 diabetes are less likely to begin labour spontaneously (19% and 34.8%, respectively) and more likely to have a caesarean birth (64.7% and 56.9%) (HQIP 2017). Monitoring and careful control of blood glucose levels between 4 and 7 mmol/L during labour may involve the use of intravenous dextrose and insulin infusions. Immediately following birth, insulin requirements are reduced, and for women with pre-existing diabetes, blood glucose monitoring will re-establish insulin requirements; for women with GDM, hypoglycaemic treatment can be discontinued (NICE 2015).

The infant

The main risks to the newborn are from hypoglycaemia or those associated with macrosomia, for instance, shoulder dystocia (Hyer & Shehata 2005). Midwives should be aware that macrosomia is more common in mothers with type 1 diabetes (18%) (HQIP 2017) and ensure that preparation for the birth involves resources for newborn life support and availability of the neonatal team. Supporting the mother with early, frequent feeding and routinely monitoring the baby's blood glucose levels can help prevent or detect neonatal hypoglycaemia (Hyer & Shehata 2005; NICE 2015) and, unless there are signs of complications, there should be no reason to separate the mother and her baby. Transfer to a neonatal unit may be necessary if the baby is or becomes unwell, for example, respiratory distress, hypoglycaemia with clinical symptoms, signs of cardiomyopathy or encephalopathy (NICE 2015). There are higher rates of term babies (28%) born to mothers with type 1 diabetes who required specialist care (HQIP 2017).

Postnatal issues

Postnatal screening of women who have had GDM leading to a diagnosis of diabetes can improve the long-term health of the mother and the outcomes of future pregnancies when maternal blood glucose levels are normalized pre-conceptually. Diagnosis may also reduce the predisposition for childhood obesity and diabetes in subsequent infants. However, the TRIAD study (Ferrara et al 2009) found that some women who had GDM did not attend for postnatal screening of diabetes. These women were more likely to have had GDM diagnosed later and were less likely to have had medical management. Ensuring that the woman's primary care team (general practitioner (GP), health visitor and practices nurses) is informed about the importance of counselling and screening might encourage women to access ongoing support and reduce women's risk after the childbearing period; coordinated efforts are important in addressing the long-term health of women with GDM and their babies.

Breastfeeding and diabetes

Women with pre-existing diabetes or GDM may be less likely to breastfeed (Much et al 2014; Sorkio et al 2010). If they do breastfeed, initiation may be delayed and the duration may be shorter, possibly on account of the increased potential for complications and interventions, such as caesarean birth (Much et al 2014; Sorkio et al 2010). Mothers with diabetes who have interventions may require additional support in the early initiation and maintenance of breastfeeding. A longitudinal study following women with GDM (Much et al 2014) showed that breastfeeding for 3 months or more was associated with a 10-year delay in the onset of type 2 diabetes when compared with women who breastfed for less than 3 months. In supporting women with GDM to breastfeed their babies, midwives can offer a low-cost intervention to reduce the risk of type 2 diabetes for the mother and their baby (Gunderson et al 2015).

Activity

What factors may make breastfeeding more challenging for women with diabetes? How can the midwife help prepare a woman with diabetes to get breastfeeding off to a good start?

Thyroid disorders

Physiological adaptations to pregnancy can mimic hyperthyroidism, although thyroid function largely remains normal. During early pregnancy, a slight fall in thyroid-stimulating hormone corresponds with increased levels of human chorionic gonadotrophin (HCG) (Karaca et al 2010; Matthews & Rankin 2017). Until the fetal thyroid begins to function at the end of the third trimester, the maternal thyroid gland is responsible for meeting maternal and fetal demands for tri-iodothyronine (T_3) and thyroxine (T_4). Abnormal levels of maternal T_4 production during this time are associated with fetal morbidity such as neurodevelopmental problems (Johansen-Bibby & Girling 2016).

Midwives are likely to be involved in providing care for women with thyroid dysfunction, although abnormal thyroid function levels can cause difficulty in conceiving or continuation of a pregnancy (Johansen-Bibby & Girling 2016). Up to 3% of childbearing-age women may be affected by thyroid problems, although most of these will have been diagnosed before pregnancy; diagnosis in pregnancy is difficult due to similarities between signs of pregnancy and thyroid dysfunction. Thyroid function levels in pregnancy differ from those of the non-pregnant population; therefore gestation-specific reference ranges should be used to interpret blood results (Johansen-Bibby & Girling 2016).

There are two main thyroid disorders: hypothyroidism and hyperthyroidism.

Hypothyroidism

Hypothyroidism affects about 20,000 pregnant women in the UK annually (Johansen-Bibby & Girling 2016). It most commonly results from an autoimmune disorder which damages the thyroid gland (Johansen-Bibby & Girling 2016). If untreated, hypothyroidism can lead to miscarriage, pre-eclampsia, anaemia, postpartum haemorrhage, preterm birth and infants of a low birth weight. Severe conditions can lead to neonatal hypothyroidism and development problems, such as attention deficit disorder (Frise & Williamson 2013; Johansen-Bibby & Girling 2016). Management aims to maintain thyroid function tests within the normal range using thyroxine replacements (for instance, levothyroxine) and monitoring levels during each trimester of pregnancy and following any changes in treatment dosage (Frise & Williamson 2013). Midwives and other health professionals can reassure women that levothyroxine can be used safely in pregnancy and lactation but should not be taken within 4 hours of iron or calcium supplements, which can interfere with absorption. If levothyroxine dosage has been increased during pregnancy, this may be reduced following pregnancy (Johansen-Bibby & Girling 2016).

Hyperthyroidism (thyrotoxicosis and Graves' disorder)

Hyperthyroidism is less common than hypothyroidism, affecting around 1 in 500 pregnancies (Frise & Williamson 2013). It presents with symptoms such as heat intolerance, tachycardia and anxiety. As with hypothyroidism, untreated women can experience miscarriage, preterm birth and fetal growth restriction (Frise & Williamson 2013), and in severe cases women can experience a thyroid storm leading to heart failure (Johansen-Bibby & Girling 2016). Treatment with anti-thyroid medication such as propylthiouracil (PTU) or carbimazole (CBZ) can normally control the disease, although where medical intervention is insufficient or the woman develops a goitre that compresses her airway, surgery may be indicated: a total or partial thyroidectomy can be performed during the second trimester of pregnancy (Johansen-Bibby & Girling 2016).

Pituitary adenoma

Pituitary adenomas account for around 10% of intracranial tumours and are associated with hypersecretion of hormones and visual and neurological impairment; the most common adenomas are clinically non-functional adenomas (CNFPAs) and prolactinomas (Zada & Carmichael 2018). The pituitary gland enlarges significantly during pregnancy and the immediate postnatal period, making it difficult to diagnose pituitary adenoma (Karaca et al 2010). However, this is more likely to have been diagnosed and treated pre-pregnancy (Johansen-Bibby & Girling 2016).

CNFPA

This type of pituitary adenoma does not present with hormonal hypersecretion (Zada & Carmichael 2018). Features include familial history of pituitary adenoma, headaches, visual field loss, erectile dysfunction in men and impaired fertility. Women with CNFPA may need treatment to reduce the tumour in order to conceive, and growth of the tumour is rare during pregnancy (Karaca et al 2010). If growth does occur, it may be treated with dopamine agonists during the third trimester (Karaca et al 2010).

Prolactinoma

Prolactinomas make up around half of functioning pituitary tumours and are relatively common in women of childbearing age (Karaca et al 2010). They are associated with amenorrhoea, anovulation infertility and galactorrhoea (production of breast milk that is unrelated to infant feeding) (Johansen-Bibby & Girling 2016), although treatment can restore fertility. Prolactin secretion is controlled by negative feedback from dopamine; therefore dopamine agonists (such as bromocriptine and cabergoline) form an important part of treatment. Small tumours (microprolactinoma) may not cause any problems and may not require treatment during pregnancy (Johansen-Bibby & Girling 2016). With larger adenomas (macroprolactinoma) couples may be advised to avoid pregnancy using non-hormonal methods of contraception until growth of the tumour has been controlled; oestrogen, used in some oral contraception, affects prolactin levels. Treatment may involve surgery or radiotherapy. During pregnancy, women require regular assessment of headaches and visual disorders. They may be prescribed dopamine agonist treatment after the first trimester to prevent further growth of the tumour, whilst minimizing the risk of teratogenicity. For some women, treatment with dopamine agonists may need to continue after birth to prevent further tumour growth. However, lactation is likely to be diminished (Frise & Williamson 2013; Karaca et al 2010). Women should be informed about the effects of treatments on lactation and may require additional support with feeding their baby.

Cushing's syndrome

Pituitary adenomas can cause high levels of cortisol (hypercortisolaemia) and are largely responsible for Cushing's syndrome. However, Cushing's syndrome is associated with infertility; therefore pregnancy is rare in women with this condition (Johansen-Bibby & Girling 2016). Adrenal disorders are responsible for around half of the cases of Cushing's syndrome in pregnancy (Karaca et al 2010).

Adrenocorticotrophic levels are high in pregnancy and at their highest during labour (Karaca et al 2010), possibly because of the physiological stress (Matthews & Rankin 2017). Resultant increases in cortisol levels during pregnancy may be responsible for the pregnancy features that resemble Cushing's syndrome (striae gravidarum, hypertension and impaired glucose tolerance). Providing a new diagnosis of Cushing's syndrome in pregnancy is therefore difficult. Pregnancy for women with Cushing's syndrome is associated with an increased chance of hypertensive disorders (70%), gestational diabetes (up to 25%), premature birth, intrauterine growth restriction and fetal death (Johansen-Bibby & Girling 2016). Multi-professional team working with endocrinologist involvement is therefore essential.

Activity

Several pregnancy-related factors make the pituitary gland vulnerable to ischaemia and necrosis (Karaca et al 2010; Matthews & Rankin 2017). Find out about Sheehan's syndrome. What is this? What is the cause, and how can it impact on women's long-term health?

Adrenal insufficiency

During pregnancy adrenal disorders are uncommon but can have a significant impact on maternal and fetal morbidity. Pregnancy makes these disorders difficult to diagnose because it can alter their presentation and, as discussed in relation to other endocrine disorders, there are common features between pregnancy and adrenal diseases (Lekarev & New 2011).

Primary adrenal insufficiency is known as *Addison's disease* and is rare during pregnancy. In the developed world it is largely an autoimmune condition with familial tendencies but is more commonly associated with tuberculosis in developing countries; other causative factors include fungal infection, haemorrhage and infarction (Lekarev & New 2011). Signs include fatigue, weight loss, dizziness and increased pigmentation of the skin (Johansen-Bibby & Girling 2016; Lerarev & New 2011). Unlike normal pregnancy changes, with Addison's disease, hyperpigmentation can occur in areas of the body that are unexposed to sunlight, for example, palmar creases and mucous membranes. Hyponatraemia is more marked than is usual for pregnancy and may cause salt cravings. When women receive appropriate treatment, pregnancy may be unproblematic, although adrenal insufficiency is associated with a small increase in preterm and caesarean births (Lerarev & New 2011).

Acute adrenal crisis can be life threatening due to significant hyponatraemia, hypotension and hypoglycaemia. Fetal production of adrenal hormones could offer some protection against such crises during pregnancy; therefore in relation to childbearing women, adrenal crisis may be more likely following birth. However, significant illness- or labour-induced stress can trigger a crisis during the third trimester (Lerarev & New 2011).

Biochemical testing involves measuring early-morning cortisol levels and synthetic adrenocorticotropic hormone (ACTH) stimulation testing; electrolyte levels may be difficult to interpret in pregnancy. Management involves multi-disciplinary team working, including endocrinologists, careful monitoring and the replacement of glucocorticoids (hydrocortisone does not cross the placenta) and mineralocorticoids throughout pregnancy. The dose is increased during periods of physiological stress, such as infection, labour or at caesarean section. Maintenance therapy of hydrocortisone following birth is safe for mothers who wish to breastfeed their babies, as breast milk transfer is very low (Lerarev & New 2011).

Activity

Pheochromocytoma is a condition that can cause pregnancy hypertension (Johansen-Bibby & Girling 2016). Find out more about this condition and the potential implications for mothers and babies. How is this diagnosed and treated?

Look back on the trigger scenario.

> *Rebecca was diagnosed with type 1 diabetes when she was 8 years old. She and her parents have always managed her diabetes carefully, following the diet, exercise and insulin therapy advised by her diabetes team. She is now 26 and in a stable relationship with Matt. They are hoping to start a family soon but are aware that there is an increased chance of complications for pregnant women with diabetes and their babies. Matt plans to attend Rebecca's next appointment with the diabetic team so that they can discuss how to avoid or minimize these potential complications.*

This scenario is one that demonstrates that some women have pre-existing endocrine disorders, such as diabetes, which can adversely affect and be affected by pregnancy. Rebecca's scenario reflects her understanding of the potential for complications and an informed, responsible attitude towards her personal and her baby's health. Now that you are familiar with diabetes in pregnancy, you should have insight into how the scenario relates to the evidence. The jigsaw model will now be used to explore the trigger scenario in more depth.

Effective communication

'Providers of pre-pregnancy advice must summarise the information given and future plans in a format that the woman can understand and keep' (Royal College of Obstetricians and Gynaecologists (RCOG) 2016:14). Furthermore, these plans should be communicated to the woman's GP and multi-disciplinary maternity care team. Questions that arise from the scenario might include: How might the effectiveness of communication regarding pre-conceptual care and childbearing be affected by involving Matt in discussions with Rebecca? How can the person discussing these issues be confident that Rebecca and Matt are able to understand and personalize this information? What methods are available for sharing plans with the GP and maternity care team?

Woman-centred care

Diabetes can affect women to varying degrees, and women's response to their condition can also differ. Plans for pre-conception, pregnancy, labour and postnatal care must be individualized according to the woman's understanding, clinical condition, lifestyle and complications. Questions arising from Rebecca's scenario might include: How can midwives keep up to date with Rebecca's plan of care? How might routine midwife appointments with Rebecca enhance the care provided by the specialist diabetic team? In what ways might reflecting on Rebecca's experiences improve midwives' ability to support other women with diabetes in pregnancy?

Using best evidence

A growing body of knowledge gained from research studies, confidential enquiries and audits relating to diabetes and pregnancy has helped improve care and outcomes for diabetic women and their babies. Questions that arise from the scenario might include: In what ways can information from the National Diabetes in Pregnancy Audit contribute to improving the experiences and outcomes of pregnant women with pre-existing diabetes? What lessons can be learned about the infants of diabetic mothers from the Confidential Enquiries into Perinatal Mortality Reports? How do the current NICE guidelines for diabetes in pregnancy compare with guidelines from other countries? How can midwives be confident that they are using the best evidence relating to diabetes in pregnancy?

Professional and legal issues

Midwives are responsible for providing safe care within a sound professional, legal and ethical framework. However, women with diabetes and their babies are at increased risk of complications and adverse outcomes. Questions that arise in relation to Rebecca's circumstances might include: Who is responsible for ensuring that midwives are equipped with the information and resources to provide safe care for women with conditions such as diabetes? How can local audits improve the experiences and outcomes of pregnancy for women with diabetes, like Rebecca? How can the midwife work within local guidelines for supporting pregnant women with diabetes whilst promoting women's autonomy?

Team working

Women with diabetes should be referred early for an appointment with a multi-disciplinary team involving obstetricians, diabetic specialists and a dietician. Questions that arise from the scenario might include: What systems are in place to ensure that women with medical conditions such as diabetes receive timely appointments with specialist teams? Is there a midwife who specializes in diabetes care where you work? What are the advantages of joint diabetes and antenatal appointments over separate appointments? How can electronic and paper documentation assist Rebecca's community midwife to act as an effective member of the multi-disciplinary team?

Clinical dexterity

It is important for pregnant women that the people providing their care are able to carry out appropriate tests to assess their own and their baby's wellbeing. Furthermore, carers must be able to recognize developing problems and respond appropriately to these (National Maternity Review 2016). Questions that arise from the scenario might include: How can the use of a customized fetal growth chart help midwives monitor fetal wellbeing? What are the signs and symptoms of hypoglycaemia and hyperglycaemia? How can these conditions be confirmed if the woman is unable to perform capillary glucose monitoring for herself? What actions should a midwife take if a woman with diabetes develops hypoglycaemia or hyperglycaemia?

Models of care

Unlike Rebecca, some women are less likely to adopt a proactive approach to their diabetic- and pregnancy-related health. These women are more likely to live in areas of socio-economic deprivation. Questions that arise in relation to the scenario could include: In what ways could care that is provided by a small team encourage women with diabetes to attend for pre-conception and antenatal care? How might care that is provided close to the woman's home improve outcomes? Why is it important to involve women with diabetes in decision-making about their pregnancy care?

Safe environment

Women and their families want access to safe maternity care, although they recognize that pregnancy and birth are not entirely free of risk (National Maternity Review 2016). Questions arising in relation to Rebecca's situation include: How can pre-conceptual and early pregnancy care from a specialist team help reduce Rebecca's risk of complications? How might multi-professional education and training improve the team's knowledge and skills relating to pregnancy care for women with diabetes? How can adverse incident reporting and reviews improve safety in clinical practice?

Promotes health

Diabetes increases the risk of complications for mothers and babies, although a number of interventions can help improve their short- and long-term health. Questions that arise from Rebecca's scenario include:

Why are HBA1c levels important in the pre-conception and early pregnancy periods? What is the reason for offering diabetic women a higher dose of folic acid? What additional assessments are offered to pregnant women with diabetes to detect developing complications? How might breastfeeding improve the long-term health of a diabetic mother and her baby?

Further scenarios

The following scenarios enable you to consider how specific situations influence the care the midwife provides. Use the jigsaw model to explore the issues raised in the scenario.

SCENARIO 1

Alice is 32 and has a history of three miscarriages. She was diagnosed with hypothyroidism 3 years ago and is currently taking medication for this. Her thyroid levels have remained within normal levels for 18 months, and she is now 7 weeks pregnant.

Practice point

Endocrine disorders can be responsible for women being unable to conceive or for early pregnancy loss.

Questions that could be asked are:
1. In what ways might Alice's previous pregnancy experiences affect her physical and emotional health in the current pregnancy?
2. What information does the midwife need to be able to provide Alice with the best information about her pregnancy?
3. How might the midwife support Alice's emotional needs during her pregnancy?
4. Who should act as the lead professional in Alice's pregnancy care?
5. How could continuity of care and carer impact on Alice's experience of pregnancy?
6. What specific conditions might Alice be at increased risk of developing as her pregnancy continues, and what is the role of the midwife in identifying and reducing the risk of harm?

SCENARIO 2

Sonia attends a booking appointment at 8 weeks' gestation. She is 28 years old, of Asian ethnic origin and has a BMI of 32. She tells you that her sister had diabetes when she was pregnant and asks whether she will develop diabetes too.

Women can present for pregnancy care with a range of characteristics that place them in a group of women who are more likely to develop gestational diabetes. Sonia has more than one factor that identifies her as being at increased risk.

Questions that could be asked are:

1. What is the role of the midwife in identifying women who are at increased risk of conditions such as gestational diabetes?
2. What investigations should the midwife offer to Sonia, and what is the ideal time for these to be performed?
3. How might sharing information with Sonia about managing gestational diabetes impact on her own, her baby's and her family's health?
4. How can high standards of documentation aid Sonia's experience and outcomes of pregnancy?
5. In what ways can specialist diabetes midwives improve the care of women who develop gestational diabetes through contact with the women themselves and by providing training for midwifery colleagues?

Conclusion

Healthy functioning of the endocrine system has a direct impact on women's ability to become pregnant, their pregnancy journey and their outcomes. Endocrine disorders therefore also have direct implications for the full range of midwifery practice: from pre-conception care, through pregnancy and birth, the postnatal period and care of the neonate, supporting mothers and babies with breastfeeding and health promotion. Through understanding about endocrine disorders and their implications for reproductive and short- and long-term health, midwives can help directly and indirectly improve the reproductive and ongoing physical, social and emotional health of these women and their families.

Resources

Diabetes UK: https://www.diabetes.org.uk/guide-to-diabetes/life-with-diabetes/pregnancy

MBRRACE-UK Perinatal Mortality Confidential Enquiry Reports: https://www.npeu.ox.ac.uk/mbrrace-uk/reports/perinatal-mortality-and-morbidity-confidential-enquiries

National Pregnancy in Diabetes (NPID) Audit: http://content.digital.nhs.uk/npid

Thyroid UK: http://www.thyroiduk.org.uk

References

Buchanan, T.A., Xiang, A., Kjos, S.L., Watanabe, R., 2007. What is gestational diabetes? Diabetes Care 30 (2), s105–s111. doi:10.2337/dc07-s201.

Ferrara, A., 2007. Increasing prevalence of gestational diabetes mellitus: a public health perspective. Diabetes Care 30 (2), s141–s146. doi:10.2337/dc07-s206.

Ferrara, A., Peng, T., Kim, C., 2009. Trends in postpartum diabetes screening and subsequent diabetes and impaired fasting glucose among women with histories of gestational diabetes mellitus: a report from the Translating Research into Action for Diabetes (TRIAD) Study. Diabetes Care 32 (2), 269–274. doi:10.2337/dc08-1184.

Frise, C.J., Williamson, C., 2013. Endocrine disease in pregnancy. Clin. Med. (Northfield Il) 13 (2), 176–181, Available at. http://www.clinmed.rcpjournal.org/content/13/2/176.full.pdf.

Gunderson, E.P., Hurston, S.R., Dewey, K.G., et al., 2015. The study of women, infant feeding and type 2 diabetes after GDM pregnancy and growth of their offspring (SWIFT Offspring study): prospective design, methodology and baseline characteristics. BMC Pregnancy Childbirth 15, 150. doi:10.1186/s12884-015-0587-z.

Health Quality Improvement Partnership (HQIP) (2017) National Pregnancy in Diabetes (NPID) Audit Report 2016. Available at: https://www.hqip.org.uk/resource/national-pregnancy-in-diabetes-audit-report-2016/.

Hyer, S.L., Shehata, H.A., 2005. Gestational diabetes mellitus. Current Obstetrics & Gynaecology 15, 368–374. doi:10.1016/j.curobgyn.2005.09.011.

International Association of Diabetes and Pregnancy Study Groups Consensus Panel, 2010. International Association of Diabetes and Pregnancy Study Groups Recommendations on the Diagnosis and Classification of Hyperglycemia in Pregnancy. Diabetes Care 33 (3), 676–682. DOI: https://doi.org/10.2337/dc09-1848.

Johansen-Bibby, A., Girling, J., 2016. Thyroid disorders and other endocrine disorders in pregnancy. Obstetrics, Gynaecology and Reproductive Medicine 26 (5), 140–148. DOI: https://doi.org/10.1016/j.ogrm.2016.02.002.

Karaca, Z., Tanriverdi, F., Unluhizarci, K., Kelestimur, F., 2010. Pregnancy and pituitary disorders. Eur. J. Endocrinol. 162, 453–475. doi:10.1530/EJE-09-0923.

Koivusalo, S.B., Rönö, K., Klemetti, M.M., et al., 2016. Gestational diabetes mellitus can be prevented by lifestyle intervention: the Finnish Gestational Diabetes Prevention Study (RADIEL): a randomized controlled trial. Diabetes Care 39, 24–30. doi:10.2337/dc15-0511.

Kourtis, A., 2012. Diabetes and gestational hypertension. Current Hypertension Reviews. 8, 127–129.

Lekarev, O., New, M.I., 2011. Adrenal disease in pregnancy. Best Practice & Research Clinical Endocrinology & Metabolism. 25, 959–973. doi:10.1016/j.beem.2011.08.004.

Lim, A.K.H. (2014) Diabetic nephropathy – complications and treatment. International Journal of Nephrology and Renovascular Disease 7: 361–381. doi:10.2147/IJNRD.S40172.

Manktelow, B.N., Smith, L.K., Prunet, C., et al. on behalf of the MBRRACE-UK Collaboration (2017) MBRRACE-UK Perinatal Mortality Surveillance Report, UK Perinatal Deaths for Births from January to December 2015. Leicester: The Infant Mortality and Morbidity Studies, Department of Health Sciences, University of Leicester. Available at: https://www.npeu. ox.ac.uk/downloads/files/mbrrace-uk/reports/MBRRACE-UK-PMS-Report-2015%20FINAL%20FULL%20REPORT.pdf.

Matthews, L., Rankin, J., 2017. The endocrine system. In: Rankin, J. (Ed.), Physiology in Childbearing With Anatomy and Related Biosciences, 4th ed. Elsevier, London, pp. 297–304.

Much, D., Beyerlein, A., Roßbauer, M., et al., 2014. Beneficial effects of breast-feeding in women with gestational diabetes mellitus. Molecular Metabolism 3 (3), 284–292. doi:10.1016/j.molmet.2014.01.002.

Murphy, H.R., 2010. Gestational diabetes: what's new? Medicine (Baltimore) 38 (12), 676–678. DOI: https://doi.org/10.1016/j.mpmed.2010.08.014.

National Institute for Health and Care Excellence (NICE) (2015) Diabetes in Pregnancy: management from pre-conception to the postnatal period. Available at: https://www.nice.org.uk/guidance/ng3.

National Maternity Review (2016) Better Births: Improving outcomes of maternity services in England. A five year forward view for maternity care. Available at: https://www.england.nhs.uk/wp-content/uploads/2016/02/national-maternity-review-report.pdf.

Rankin, J., 2017. Diabetes mellitus and other metabolic disorders in pregnancy. In: Rankin, J. (Ed.), Physiology in Childbearing With Anatomy and Related Biosciences, 4th ed. Elsevier, London, pp. 361–370.

Royal College of Obstetricians and Gynaecologists (2016) Providing Quality Care for Women. A framework for maternity service standards. Available at: https://www.rcog.org.uk/globalassets/documents/guidelines/working-party-reports/maternitystandards.pdf.

Sorkio, S., Cuthbertson, D., Bärlund, S., et al. TRIGR Study Group, 2010. Breastfeeding patterns of mothers with type 1 diabetes: results from an infant feeding trial. Diabetes & Metabolic Syndrome: Clinical Research & Reviews 26, 206–211. doi:10.1002/dmrr.1074.

Starikov, R., Dudley, D., Reddy, U.M., 2015. Stillbirth in the pregnancy complicated by diabetes. Curr. Diab. Rep. 15, 11. doi:10.1007/s11892-015-0580-y.

Whitelaw, B., Gayle, C., 2010. Gestational diabetes. Obstetrics, Gynaecology and Reproductive Medicine 21 (2), 41–46. DOI: https://doi.org/10.1016/j.ogrm.2010.11.001.

Zada, G., Carmichael, J. (2018) Pituitary adenoma. BMJ Best Practice. Available at: https://bestpractice.bmj.com/topics/en-gb/1030.

Page numbers followed by '*f*' indicate figures, '*t*' indicate tables, and '*b*' indicate boxes.